Getting It Together!

*Your Self-paced
Cellulite and Love-handle
Fitness Solution*

Published by:

John Ireland
401 Manhattan Beach Blvd.
Manhattan Beach, CA
U.S.A.

All rights reserved.   No part of this book may be reproduced or transmitted in any form or by any means, electronic or mechanical, including photocopying, recording, or by information storage and retrieval system without written permission from the author, except for the inclusion of brief quotations in a review.

Copyright 1994 by John Ireland
Printed in the United States of America

Library of Congress Cataloging-in-Publication Data

Ireland, John Edge, 1951-
Getting it together!

Bibliography: p.
Includes index.
1. Physical fitness. 2. Exercise. I. Title.

ISBN 0-9641202-5-9 (soft)

For Coach Ed Franz, Physical Education instructor, San Diego State University:

Here's the final version of that rough draft I submitted as a paper in your class ...

Contents

Foreword by Lyle Alzado 7
    Endorsements by: 8
Periodical Reviews: 18
About This Book 35
Acknowledgements 37
Chapter 1: First, Some Fitness Mythology **39**
Chapter 2: Getting Started **49**
    Evaluate How Your Body Currently Operates 50
    Evaluate Your Body's Current Appearance 50
    Where Are You Going From Here? 51
    How Are You Going To Get There? 51
Chapter 3: About Your Eating Habits **53**
    Two Simple Rules 54
    Why Complex Carbohydrates Are Encouraged 54
    Why Fats Are To Be Avoided 54
    A Few Other Things To Avoid 55
    What About Proteins? 55
    Vitamins and Minerals 56
    A Few More "Do's" and "Don'ts" 57
Chapter 4: Your Exercise Program; The Schedule **63**
    Step 1: Select Specific Exercises 64
        For Strengthening/Maintaining Cardiorespiratory System: 65
    Step 2: Devise Your Workout Schedule 66
        List "Your" Exercises On Separate Sheets of Paper 66
        Categorize the Exercises 67
            Separate Upper Body Exercises From Lower Body Exercises ... 67
            Separate De-Massing Exercises From Building Exercises 67
        Assign Exercises To Specific Days 68
            Include Sufficient Aerobic Exercise In Your Schedule 68
            Recommended outdoor aerobics: 69
            Recommended indoor aerobics: 69
            Follow Recommended Session Minimums and Maximums 70
            Order Exercises According to Muscle Sizes Involved 70
            Allow Time In Each Session For Stretching 70
            Include Time For Enjoying the Post-Workout Glow 71
    Devising (and Revising) a Schedule: an Example 71
    Step 3: Follow the Program 75
        Breathe Properly 75

Getting It Together: Introduction

Keep Your Stomach Pulled In 75
Exercise To Proper "Fatigue Level" 76
Warm Up To Each Exercise 76
Don't Exceed Recommended Maximums 76
Perform Aerobic Exercises Properly 76
    Determine Your Proper Heart Rate For Aerobic Exercise 77
    Monitor Your Heart Rate 78
    Heart Rate Equivalency Chart 79

Chapter 5. Water Routines: Aerobic Exercises For De-Massing; Strengthening Cardiorespiratory System 81
    "Well, That All Makes Sense and Sounds Very Fine, But ..." 82
    "... I Don't Have a Swimming Pool" 82
    "... I'm Not a Swimmer" or "... I Can't (or Don't Want to) Get My Head Wet" 82
How to Perform Water Routines 83
    For de-massing the upper body 84
    For de-massing the lower body 85
    For maintaining the target area 86
        BREAST STROKE (Arms Only) 86
        AUSTRALIAN CRAWL (Arms Only) 88
        BACKSTROKE (Arms Only) 90
        FLUTTER KICKS (Legs Only) 92
        FROG KICKS (Legs Only) 94
        STANDING KNEE LIFTS (Legs Only) 96
        STANDING FROG KICKS (Legs Only) 97

Chapter 6: Weight Room Routines; Anaerobic Exercises for Increasing, Strengthening Selected Muscles 99
How to Work With Weights 100
    For building the target area 100
    For toning the target area 102
    For maintaining the target area 102
        SHOULDER SHRUGS 103
        MILITARY PRESSES 104
        FLAT BENCH PULLOVER 105
        FLAT BENCH PRESSES 107
        INCLINE BENCH PRESSES 108
        DECLINE BENCH PRESSES 109
        BEHIND-THE-NECK PULL DOWNS 111
        PRESS DOWNS 112
        SUPPORTED CURLS 113
        WEIGHTED SIT BACKS 115
        WEIGHTED THREE-QUARTER SQUATS 116

Getting It Together: Introduction

  LEG CURLS 118
  WEIGHTED CALF RAISES 119
Chapter 7: Floor Exercises; Aerobic or Anaerobic Exercises For Maintenance, At-Home Substitutes **121**
 How To Perform Floor Exercises 122
  For Maintenance 122
  As Substitutes For Water or Weight Room Routines 122
  For Aerobic Value 122
   ARM TWIRLS 123
   SHOULDER SHRUGS 124
   CHIN UPS 125
   PUSH UPS - 1 127
   PUSH UPS - 2 128
   SIT BACKS 130
   HIP RAISES 131
   THREE-QUARTER SQUATS 132
   LEG LIFTS 134
   CALF RAISES 135
Appendix **137**
 Recommended Reading 137
 About the Author 137
  A Page From John's Photo Album 140
 Index 143

Foreword by Lyle Alzado

Listen up. I'm a professional football player. I work for a guy whose motto is "committment to excellence." My job is to go upside the heads of people whose job it is to go upside my head. Despite a fairly constant ringing between my ears and a somewhat uneven disposition I've been pretty good at my job for years.

The reason I'm good is that I always stay in great shape. Being big and a little unpredictable helps too but that's not the point as far as you're concerned. After all, you may not want to be a professional football player. All you want is to find an easy-as-pie way to get in great shape so you can look good and feel good.

Which brings us to the subject of this book. My friend John Ireland who wrote this book swears that his system for getting you in great shape is better than any other system because it's easy as pie. John, of course, is as full of it as the next guy whose main goal is to sell a lot of books.

Face it. Getting in great shape is hard stinking work no matter how you do it. You gotta eat right and you gotta work out regular, both of which are very hard to do.

The real reason John's system is better than any other I've run across is that it is straightforward and complete. You get the right information about the basic elements of physical fitness, namely proper diet and regular helpings of the right kinds of exercise. Plus, you learn how to set up your very own fitness program to achieve your very own personal goals at your very own pace.

The bottom line is this: John's book, like no other I've seen, tells you how to become your own physical fitness boss and encourages you to make your own personal "committment to excellence."

Now get outta my face. We got some sweating to do.

Lyle Alzado
Manhattan Beach, 1985

P.S. Say no to steroids!

Endorsements by:

Jim Anderson
Trainer
Los Angeles Rams

Scott Morrison
Trainer
Los Angeles Lazers

Gary Vitti
Trainer
 Los Angeles Lakers

Bill Buhler
Head Trainer
Los Angeles Dodgers

George Anderson and Rod Martin
Trainers
Los Angeles Raiders

Pete Demers
Trainer
Los Angeles Rams

George H. Allen
Chairman and CEO
National Fitness Foundation
(former Head Coach Los Angeles Rams and Washington Redskins)

Ken Locker
Physical Trainer
Dallas Cowboys

Every avenue of Getting It Together! meets with my approval. It's excellent at helping the reader set goals, it describes a wide variety of easy-to-understand exercises, and it offers good guidelines for assessing improvements. The tips on food consumption are the same ones I've been recommending for years.

And although John makes it clear that you don't have to have your own swimming pool to make use of his new routines for eliminating unwanted fat, anyone who *does* have a pool will be delighted to find a practical use for it.

This is a great book for the amateur/weekend athlete who doesn't have access to professional training facilities. Getting It Together! is a well-rounded source of information for all active individuals and can help them achieve top physical condition.

Jim Anderson
Trainer, Los Angeles Rams

Anyone who wants to get into shape — or *back* into shape — should have Getting It Together! It provides a sound foundation which you can then temper to suit your individual needs. Pro athletes such as our players, for example, can increase the intensity of the routines, while a novice might start with less intense workouts.

I was particularly pleased to come across an idea I've always held to be true but which I'd never before seen so convincingly stated and justified: that a mirror is a far better tool than a scale for measuring your progress.

Getting It Together! gives you good information and it's easy to read and understand. In a word, the book is clean.

Scott Morrison
Trainer, Los Angeles Lazers

As the trainer of the Los Angeles Lakers, I read numerous articles and books regarding physical fitness and nutrition. There's certainly no shortage of literature currently available on these subjects; unfortunately, the "information" presented in some of them is so off-base it's actually frightening. Getting It Together! is clearly written and easy to follow and I recommend it for the novice trying to improve his or her fitness level.

Gary Vitti
Trainer, Los Angeles Lakers

How did I like John Ireland's new fitness book? Enough to recommend it to *all* my friends — including one particular bunch of guys who will be "Getting It Together!" under my supervision next spring.

Bill Buhler
Head Trainer, Los Angeles Dodgers

Getting It Together! proves that you don't need expensive health spas or exotic clinics to learn how to get in shape — you can be creative and design our own program! It also provides the true answer, the healthy alternative, to diet pills.

Simple to read, the book takes a down to earth approach to fitness and leads you step by step. It gives you a clear idea of what can be accomplished and of what to look for in terms of improvements.

George Anderson and Rod Martin
Trainers, Los Angeles Raiders

I've never before read a fitness book that kept me wanting to turn the pages, but I did with Getting It Together! The information is so clear, interestingly presented, and precise without getting bogged down in overly technical details that I read it straight through.

It supports ideas and techniques we teach our players, but this book is suitable for virtually anyone: people with no current fitness program as well as professional athletes. I especially recommend it to amateur athletes just getting started because it will teach them correct ways to eat and exercise and (at least equally importantly) some common incorrect ways.

Pete Demers
Trainer, Los Angeles Kings

If you're not in shape everything is too much work. John Ireland's new book, Getting It Together!, offers fitness fundamental adults can use to map out their own personal fitness game plan. What are you waiting for? Get fit!

George H. Allen
Chairman and CEO,
National Fitness Foundation
Former Head Coach, Los Angeles Rams
Former Head Coach, Washington Redskins

Here's a well-organized common sense approach to the fitness craze — not just a make-over. Amateur athletes and individuals can use Getting It Together! as an overall fitness conditioning program guide.

Ken Locker
Physical Trainer, Dallas Cowboys

Periodical Reviews:

In addition to the endorsements previously listed, this book has been reviewed by a number of prestigious periodicals as shown below in the "As featured in . . ." section below.

As Featured in ...
P.A.T.S
Professional Athletic Therapy Services, Inc.

I have recently had the opportunity to review Getting It Together! Your Personal Self-Paced Fitness Program For Maximum Results and found it to be quite interesting and informative. The general fitness principles and individual exercise descriptions are well presented and clearly written. This book is a great way to get the average individual going with a well designed exercise program — especially for "demassing."

In short, I found the book worthwhile reading and I would not hesitate to recommend it to someone looking to begin a fitness program.

Dave Harding
Athletic therapist

As featured in...
HEALTHFUL Living

Volume V, No. 5

Book Reviews

Ireland believes that before beginning a fitness program, you must do three things: assess your body, define your goals and design a program that will help you realize those goals. Approximately half of the book is devoted to describing and illustrating the specific exercises and routines that should make up a good fitness plan. The routines fall into 3 categories: water routines, weight lifting and floor exercises.

Ireland also takes the time to dispel some commonly believed fitness myths and discusses a few simple guidelines to eating correctly. The main emphasis of his book, though, is to enable the reader to assess the current state of his/her body, define the things that need to be changed and devise an exercise program that is custom-tailored to achieving those objectives in the most efficient manner possible.

Ireland provides solid information for those who wish to embark on a fitness program but don't know where to begin. The exercises are described thoroughly and are illustrated clearly. Routines are aimed at "de-massing," building up, or maintaining. This book is highly recommended as providing a good starting point for implementing an exercise program.

As featured in...
IDEAS FOR BETTER LIVING
August 1986   Vol. 5, No. 1

The Bookshelf

None of the conventional types of exercise — running, jogging, swimming laps, aerobic dancing, lifting weights, and so on — can produce all of the results you seek from an exercise program, according to author Ireland.

The book presents new techniques and a new approach to fitness, an approach Lyle Alzado describes in his Foreword as "straightforward and complete."

Ireland recognizes that no one fitness program can be right for everyone. Instead, he leads the reader through a step-by-step procedure for designing his or her own exercise program, from assessing the current situation, pinpointing areas needing change, defining exact goals, and selecting appropriate exercises, to combining those exercises into a personal workout routine.

The book describes and illustrates an entirely new set of routines developed by the author for eliminating unwanted fat, the weight room routines he has found most effective for building and strengthening individual areas, and selected floor exercises for maintenance or "at-home" substitutes.

Because the exercises themselves are the most efficient at what they do, and because each person controls his or her own schedule, the result is an exercise program that's custom-tailored to achieving that person's fitness goals in the most convenient, efficient manner possible.

Ireland also explains why carbohydrates are not the enemy — and why fats are — and offers easy-to-follow guidelines on how to modify eating habits to complement the exercise program.

As featured in...
SOUTHERN CALIFORNIA'S RUNNING & TRIATHLON NEWS

"Getting It Together"

"Getting It Together," by John Edge Ireland is what you might call your complete fitness book. It has exercises and programs to help you firm up, limber up and strengthen up. He offers a whole series of water routines, weight routines and stretching routines. Plus, best of all, it's written in a manner that makes it enjoyable reading. "Getting It Together" makes a great resource book, no matter what your fitness level. Lyle Alzado, the former Los Angeles Raider lineman, sums up the book this way in his foreword: "The bottom line is this: John's book, like no other I've seen, tells you how to become your own personal fitness boss and encourages you to make your own personal 'commitment to excellence.' Now get outta my face...we got some sweating to do."

Personally, I try not to argue with men the size of Vermont. I think you'll enjoy the book.

As featured in...
SCOTTISH DIVER

Book Reviews

I had but a moment of hesitation before accepting this book for review. Some divers think that fitness programmes are far removed from their needs. How wrong they are! It's quite clear from our Training Manual that fitness is important. Getting it together is about the regaining, maintaining and development of fitness. It's primarily oriented towards aerobic exercise in the swimming pool together with aerobic weightlifting routines. This emphasis on pool work should make it especially interesting to divers. In other respects the book can be described as a sensible and balanced account of methods of exercise which may make you slimmer and stronger and are almost certain to make you fitter.

Adam Curtis

As featured in...
SKI SURVEY
BRITAIN'S LARGEST CERTIFIED CIRCULATION SKI MAGAZINE

TITLES

If you are not satisfied with the shape of your body, Getting it Together by John Edge Ireland will be your Bible. Written by an American in typically chatty style, it is riveting. It gives you all the information for putting together a personal exercise programme. The workouts range through stretch, aerobic and strengthening carried out on the floor, in the pool or at the gym. Illustrations show muscle groups used. He dispels several myths and has fascinating new theories. There is even a log book to monitor progress. It is the author's personal experience, enthusiastically shared with us. It would suit someone starting out or dissatisfied with a routine. Although not specific to skiing it has a place as a programme planned for year round ski fitness.

As featured in...
PERSONAL VITALITY

**Your Fitness
December 1989**

Good News About Health, Wealth and Happiness

John Edge Ireland

Getting it Right:
Fitness Myths Debunked

Are you still out of shape, even though you've been dieting and exercising? If so, you probably don't have your facts about fitness quite right.

So suggests John Edge Ireland, author of Getting it Together: Your Personal Self-Paced Fitness Program For Maximum Results. "Nobody has definitive answers to all the questions about how to best get fit. There's plenty of room for plenty of theories, and there's been no shortage of theorists eager to supply ready answers. Their answers range from the reasonable to the ridiculous, and as a result, lots of misinformation and misconceptions surround the subject of fitness," Ireland says.

In working out, you may be following one of the fitness myths mentioned below. If so, now is the time to set yourself straight and get yourself on the right track.

FITNESS MYTHS

All it takes is eating right and plenty of exercise. This statement isn't inaccurate, but it is incomplete. You need to get plenty of the right kind of exercise; that is, exercise that won't injure your joints and ligaments and that provides a complete cardiovascular workout.

The very best form of exercise for staying in shape is _____. Even though there's plenty of answers you can give — running, aerobic dancing, swimming, weight lifting, etc. — the fact is, there is no one single form of exercise that is best for everyone. Rather, in most cases, the most effective,

Getting It Together: Introduction

time-efficient fitness program involves two forms of exercise — one that provides an aerobic workout (jogging, for example), and one that calls for isolation exercises to develop strength (weight training, for example).

Spot reducing can remove fat selectively. This principle seems logical enough. If you want to get rid of a particular bulge of fat, doesn't it stand to reason that exercising that area would burn it off?

No. The truth is, external approaches don't work. Vibrating or jiggling fat doesn't make it go away. And devices like sweat suits, saunas or inflated belts or pants leave the fat undisturbed. Yes, you will lose body fluids (in the form of sweat), but the losses will be temporary. And as soon as the lost fluids are replaced, any reduced areas assume their original sizes.

Your weight is the truest measure of your progress. A scale indicates the total amount of weight placed on it, but not the distribution of that weight. A mirror gives a much better indication of the shape your body is in. It shows the areas that are out of shape, letting you see where you need to concentrate your efforts.

Remember: Muscle outweighs fat by 2-to-1. If you remove fat from your body and improve muscle tone at the same time, you may actually see a net gain in weight when you step on your scale. Look in the mirror, however, and you will see a stronger, trimmer and more attractive you.

As some people get older, they stay overweight no matter what they do. It is true that many people become (and remain) overweight as they get older, but their excess weight is not due to some unavoidable trick of fate. What actually happens is quite simple: As some people get older, they gradually tend to grow away from the physically demanding activities of their younger years — without adjusting their eating habits accordingly. The inevitable? The same caloric intake with less calories burned equals fat.

I don't have time to exercise. Vast amounts of time are not required to get fit and stay that way. If your fitness program is properly designed, it will give you the results you seek in the minimum time possible because it will be focused precisely and exclusively on your objectives. You can expect to attain results by spending as little as 20 minutes, three times a week in a regular workout.

As featured in...
SCHOLASTIC COACH

Incorporating ATHLETIC Journal
October 1987
PUBLISHED BY SCHOLASTIC, INC.
VOL. 57, No. 3

NEW BOOKS

FITNESS

(A Personal fitness guide that tells you simply and soundly how to devise an all around exercise program. The book is exceptionally clear and readable, with a super chapter on fitness mythology and sections on eating habits, water routines, weight-room routines, and floor exercises. We found it interesting and persuasive.)

As featured in...
WORLD ACROBATICS

Vol. 10, Number 11

BOOK REVIEW

'Getting it Together' by John Edge Ireland is a well put together volume easy to follow with nice diagrams, a book for those who are health and fitness conscious. It offers suggestions and points of view for those who are already on their own style of programme and those who seek to improve their fitness. From the material in the pages anyone with a desire to achieve physical improvement can put together their own programme to suit their lifestyle and motivation.

As featured in...
SWIMMING POOL AGE SPA MERCHANDISER

Fitness Book

New techniques and a new approach to fitness are presented in a new book by John Edge Ireland called "Getting it Together! Your Personal Self-Paced Fitness Program for Maximum Results."

Ireland leads the reader through a step-by-step procedure for designing his or her own exercise program, including assessing the current situation, pinpointing areas needing change, defining exact goals, selecting appropriate exercises and combining those exercises into a personal workout routine.

The 160-page book describes and illustrates a set of routines developed by the author for eliminating unwanted fat, the weight-room routines he has found most effective for building and strengthening individual areas and selected floor exercises for maintenance or "at-home substitutes."

As featured in...
Jack Hutslar's SPORT SCENE

This book is your personal self-paced fitness programs for maximum results. The author, a physical educator, discusses fitness mythology, and there is a lot of it in ads on the tube, getting started, eating habits, exercise schedules, aerobic exercises so important for cardiovascular fitness, weight room stuff and floor exercises you can do at home.

The book is well illustrated so the exercise gymnologist knows what muscle group is doing the work. Ireland also included a dozen handy work out schedules to help you stay on task. No pain! No gain!

Jack Hutslar, PhD
NAYSI NEWS, INFORMATION AND RESOURCE CENTER
North American Youth Sport Institute
Kernersville, NC

As featured in...
ATHLETIC Journal

The thesis is that you can design your own effective fitness program. You get advice on how to trim it down, build it up and/or improve its functioning. The various recommended land and water exercises are unique in that accompanying drawings depict both the "do" and the "don't." An appendix contains 13 detailed workout schedule forms. The author, a three-sport school athlete and physical education graduate, is a "civilian" practitioner of the book's concepts. He cites as myths that carbohydrates are fattening, that spot reducing can remove fat selectively, that women become over muscular if they lift weights and that older people stay overweight no matter what they do.

As featured in...
The Small Press Book Review

Getting It Together does not present a particular program of exercise for improving or maintaining appearance and health. This makes it different from most other books on exercising. What it does is give information and advice so that the reader can devise his own regimen of exercise to reach particular aims he has. These aims may be general, such as maintaining good muscle tone overall or keeping up cardiovascular fitness; or they may be specific, such as flattening one's stomach or building up the strength in one's legs. The book is especially pertinent for reaching specific aims.

John Ireland has a degree in physical education from San Diego State University (CA). He devised the many-faceted and changeable program for exercise explained in his Getting It Together when he wasn't getting the results he wanted after following commonly accepted tips and practices for staying in shape and reaching particular goals. There are three broad aims in Ireland's approach — de-massing, i.e., getting rid of fat and improving muscle tone; enlarging and strengthening muscles; and maintaining the result(s) one has achieved. Within each of these broad aims of exercising, there are the related specific aims of shedding fat from thighs, strengthening shoulders, keeping the stomach flat, etc. The reader chooses his own goal; and then using charts, illustrations, instructions, and general commentary, he designs the program that will bring him to it. The exercises recommended and described are mostly water exercises, ones that make use of moderate weights, and light calisthenics, varying depending on the reader's goal.

Ireland also gives general information and advice on proper eating, maintaining health, and beginning and adhering to an exercise program. He tells the reader how to evaluate his present physical condition; what to consider in choosing aims and outlining a program; and how to achieve the aims selected. The illustrations showing the various exercises, pointing out the muscles involved in them and in some cases showing what shouldn't be done if an exercise is to serve its purposes, make it easy for the reader to devise the exercise program suited to his aims. Getting It Together comes with a brief "Foreword" by the football player Lyle Alzado.

As featured in...
The Paris Post-Intelligencer

Tee Pee talks
By TOMMY PRIDDY

I finished reading a book on physical fitness which would be a tremendous help to anyone currently working out or thinking of getting in shape.

The book is Getting It Together! Your Personal Self-Paced Fitness Program For Maximum Results by John Edge Ireland. Ireland has produced a book describing new water-related exercises, weight training, floor exercises and eating habits.

Ireland's key to successfully getting physically fit is self-assessment. He advises the readers to take a look at themselves and evaluate what needs to be done. After deciding what needs to be worked on, he tells the readers, they need to decide on a course of action that best suits their needs and time requirements.

The book is written in an entertaining manner the reader will be able to relate to when deciding to begin a workout program. Diagrams and charts are included.

Those planning to begin a workout program or wanting to get better results from the one they are currently using, I'd recommend reading this book.

As featured in...
THE TENNISPRO
Official Publication of the U.S. Professional Tennis Registry Foundation

Book Review
"Getting It Together"

None of the conventional types of exercise — running, jogging, swimming laps, aerobic dancing, lifting weights, and so on — can produce all of the results you seek from an exercise program.

So asserts John Edge Ireland in his new book Getting It Together!

The book presents new techniques and a new approach to fitness, an approach Lyle Alzado describes in his Foreword as "straightforward and complete."

Ireland recognizes that no one fitness program can be right for everyone. Instead, he leads the reader through a step-by-step procedure for designing his or her own exercise program, from assessing the current situation, pinpointing areas needing change, defining exact goals, and selected appropriate exercises, to combining those exercises into a personal workout routine.

The book describes and illustrates an entirely NEW set of routines developed by the author for eliminating unwanted fat like cellulite and "love handles," the weight room routines he has found most effective for building and strengthening individual areas, and selected floor exercises for maintenance or "at-home" substitutes.

Because the exercises themselves are the most efficient at what they do, and because each person controls his or her own schedule, the result is an exercise program that's custom tailored to achieving that person's fitness goals in the most convenient, efficient manner possible.

As featured in...
AAA SPOTLIGHT

March 1990

When it comes to good health
and fit bodies, it's either hit or myth.

You diet, you exercise. But a few flights of stairs winds you, and you still don't have the firm body you know that you could have. What's going on?

According to John Edge Ireland, author of Getting it Together: Your Personal Self-Paced Fitness Program for Maximum Results, fitness is fraught with "misinformation and misconceptions" that could hinder your progress. They include:

Myth: All it takes is eating right and plenty of exercise.

Fact: This statement isn't complete. You need to get plenty of the right kind of exercise, exercise that won't injure your joints and ligaments and that provides a complete cardiovascular workout.

Myth: Your weight is the truest measure of your progress.

Fact: A scale indicates your total weight, but not the distribution of that weight. A mirror is a better indicator of the shape your body is in than a scale. Muscle outweighs fat 2-to-1. If you remove fat from your body and improve muscle tone at the same time, you may actually see a net gain in weight. In the mirror, however, you'll see a trimmer, stronger, more attractive body.

Myth: Spot reducing can remove fat selectively.

Fact: External approaches don't work. Vibrating or jiggling fat doesn't make it go away. Sweat suits, saunas, inflated belts or pants leave fat undisturbed. You lose only water weight which is only temporary.

Myth: The very best form of exercise is _____.

Fact: There is no single form of exercise that is best for everyone. In

Getting It Together: Introduction

most cases, the most effective time-efficient fitness program involves two forms of exercise — aerobic, and isolation exercises for strength (weights, for example).

Myth: As some people get older, they stay overweight no matter what they do.

Fact: While some people become and remain overweight as they get older, their fat is not due to some trick of fate. Older people tend to grow less active without adjusting their eating habits. The inevitable happens.

Myth: I don't have time to exercise.

Fact: You can expect to attain results by exercising as little as 20 minutes, three times a week. If your fitness program is properly designed, it will give you the results you seek in the minimum time possible because it will be focused exclusively to your objectives.

About This Book ...

The true key to "getting it together" — to achieving the look and feel you seek — is to define a fitness program that works for *you*, one that achieves *your* goals.

It's unrealistic to expect that anyone will read a book, make drastic changes in his or her life style, and then maintain those changes for any meaningful length of time. This book was written with no such expectations and makes no such demands of you. You'll find no prescribed exercise or diet plan with hard-and-fast rules (complete with descriptions of the dire consequences you'll face if you'll break them). No single exercise/diet plan can be right for everyone.

What you *will* find in this book are some simple general guidelines about your eating habits and a straightforward step-by-step procedure for designing your own exercise program.

You start by assessing your current state of fitness and defining your goals. Next, you select individual exercises aimed at each area you want to work, either to "de-mass" it (i.e., to eliminate unwanted fat while improving muscle tone) and strengthen your cardiorespiratory system, build muscle size and strength, or maintain the area's current status. You then combine those exercises into your personal workout routine, scheduled to fit most conveniently with your other activities.

This book details a number of specific exercises, some performed in water (for de-massing and strengthening your cardiorespiratory system), some with weights (for building), and others as floor exercises (for maintaining or as substitutes when you can't get to the water or weight room). Each is the most effective I've found at isolating and concentrating effort on "its" area.

Because the exercises themselves are the most efficient at what they do, and because you control the schedule, the result is an exercise program that's custom-tailored to achieving your objectives in the most convenient, efficient manner possible.

However, a fitness program will work for you only if it becomes a part of your life. It's not enough to define an eating and exercise program targeted to your specific objectives; that program must also be one you'll actually follow. And what better way to increase the odds of finding a program you'll stick with than to design that program yourself?

Acknowledgements

A lot of people helped make this book possible, and I'd like to thank a few of them here.

Ed Franz, to whom this book is dedicated, for his patience and understanding, and for pointing out that there are careers other than in professional sports.

Jim Shaw, for recommending:
Publitec Editions as a publisher.

Yvette Hamby, for recommending:
Joe Yule as an illustrator.

Larry Petrill, former football coach, Aviation High School (Manhattan Beach, California), and current assistant football coach, San Jose State University, for giving me my first lessons in training and fitness.

Bea Cottington, Linda Meier, and Erik Fair, for their insightful reviews and helpful comments.

Diana Lipson, R.D. THE ENERGY RESOURCE, for her insightful review and helpful comments.

Dr. Dennis A. Nowack, The Manhattan Beach Chiropractic Center, for his helpful comments.

Rod Stafford, for his help with the cover design and production.

John Post, for his cover photographs.

Phil Callihan, for recommending:
Allan Kidd for page design and layup.

Chapter 1: First, Some Fitness Mythology

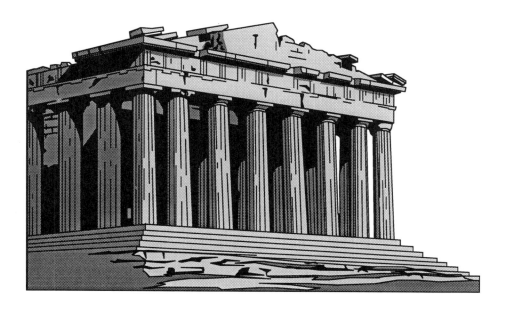

Nobody has definitive answers to all the questions about the human body and how it can "best" be brought to (and kept in) a state of physical fitness. There's plenty of room for plenty of theories, and there's been no shortage of theorists eager to supply ready answers. Their answers have ranged from the reasonable to the ridiculous, and as a result, lots of misinformation and misconceptions surround the subject of fitness.

Before we get started, let's clear the air of at least some of the most persistent of these myths.

Myth #1:
"All It Takes Is Eating Right and Plenty of Exercise"

Actually, this statement isn't so much inaccurate as it is incomplete. If it urged you to get plenty of the *right kind* of exercise, I'd have no argument with it whatsoever.

Just what is the right kind of exercise? Well, there are lots of ready answers to that one, too ...

Myth #2:
"The Very Best Form of Exercise For Staying In Shape Is ..."

...Gross Aerobic Exercise

Exercises like jogging, running, aerobic dancing, jumping jacks, or skipping rope involve the entire body (hence the "gross") and are intensely aerobic in nature. (Swimming is also a gross aerobic exercise, but we'll consider that shortly.)

That is, gross aerobic exercise does an excellent job of elevating your heart rate and intensifying your breathing. These forms of exercise, if done properly, are undeniably effective in lowering your heart rate and building your stamina. When done at the correct level, they also promote the creation of enzymes in the muscles which enhance the muscles' ability to burn fat efficiently while simultaneously creating the caloric demand necessary for the body's stored resources (fat) to be called upon.

There are, however, a number of major, well-documented drawbacks to gross aerobic exercise. The continuous pounding can (and often does) result in tendinitis, torn ligaments, stress fractures, and various forms of damage to the spine, knees, ankles, and feet, in various degrees of severity. What effect do you suppose all that up-and-down pounding has on your face? Doesn't it make sense that it could only accelerate gravity's aging effect?

As one wit put it, such exercise does at least four things to your body ... and one of those things is good. There's yet another drawback. While gross aerobic exercise may do a good job of keeping you *in* shape from a cardio-respiratory standpoint, it isn't so effective at making selected improvements in the shape *of* your shape.

Gross aerobic exercise works all of the body simultaneously, which means that no individual area is exercised with maximum efficiency. People using this type of exercise in an attempt to change their outward appearance too often find that they've lost in areas they wanted to increase, while the areas they wanted to reduce seem to have increased! (Actually, these areas have probably remained the same, but appear larger because the surrounding areas have decreased.)

The reason for this phenomenon is quite straightforward. Large muscle groups such as the thigh and buttock muscles can withstand far more exertion before altering their resting states than can small muscle groups like those of the arms, shoulders, neck, and face. Therefore, the small muscle groups always fatigue before the large muscle groups.

This phenomenon is revealed perhaps most dramatically in the bodies of "real" runners, people to whom running is a way of life. Runners regularly exert the large muscle groups of their lower bodies to, and often beyond, the point of fatigue. The smaller muscle groups of their upper bodies, meanwhile, participate throughout the total effort, which means that those muscles are routinely exerted far beyond the point of fatigue. The result is that runners develop strong, lean lower body muscles and their upper bodies thin out.

Many of the characteristics of a "runner's body" are highly desirable. Who doesn't want a strong heart, terrific stamina, and a metabolism that's better geared to burning fat than it is to storing it? Not everyone especially wants to *look* like a runner, however. Many people prefer a more solid, more muscular body; others aim for a smoother, firmer look. Such goals simply can't be achieved with a program of running, jogging, aerobic dancing, swimming, or similar exercises alone.

The bottom line is this: gross aerobic exercise is highly effective at building stamina and improving muscle metabolism, but in every other way it's either inherently harmful or potentially damaging to your body. And, unless your goal is to have a "runner's body," it won't produce the changes in your appearance you may be seeking. Every fitness program should include sufficient aerobic exercise, but in a more positive form.

... Swimming Laps

Some people say, "If you're going to do just one type of exercise, you should swim laps." I agree. Swimming probably *is* the most beneficial single type of exercise overall. It provides the aerobic value of other forms of gross aerobic exercise without many of the associated drawbacks.

Unfortunately, swimming does share one major drawback: it isn't effective for achieving specific changes in how you look because it isn't efficient at exercising individual parts of your body. Because you use virtually all parts of your body in swimming, the effort extracted from any one particular area is diluted.

The bottom line here is that swimming would be a better choice than other gross aerobics *if* you were forced to limit yourself to one form of exercise ... but it still isn't the complete answer if you want to modify how your body looks.

... Lifting Weights

Many people regard weight lifting as a panacea, a sure-fire way to achieve any fitness goal you could possibly have.

I confess that I used to be a true believer. For years, I accepted this myth in its entirety, and couldn't understand why I wasn't getting *all* the results I was seeking. Try as I might, the "love handles," protruding belly and buttocks, and heavy legs still followed me into the mirror.

Looking around for a solution, I considered the swimming pool at my gym. I knew that doctors had been recommending water as a therapeutic medium for years. (Because of the support water provides, patients can rehabilitate muscles without stressing joints.) I had read that water provides 12 times as much resistance as air, and I knew from experience that moving through water offers tremendous aerobic value.

All in all, swimming looked like a great way to eliminate those stubborn areas of excess fat, except that it also looked like a pretty inefficient way to go about it. So much of the work involved in swimming comes from the arms, shoulders, and back, areas I wasn't trying to de-mass.

The upshot was that I worked out an exercise I can perform in a swimming pool to take advantage of the water's supportive nature and all that extra resistance, but which concentrates the effort on the areas I *was* trying to de-mass. And it worked! My body finally looks the way I've always wanted. (Since then, I've expanded on that first exercise and developed a set of water routines that are the best way I've found for getting rid of unwanted fat. But I'm getting ahead of myself.)

Conclusion: As good as the weight room is for accomplishing a wide variety of objectives, it isn't always the answer either.

Then what is the answer?

The way around these problems is, in the briefest possible terms, twofold: aerobic exercise of a positive, non-destructive nature, and isolation exercises for intensive, concentrated work on individual areas of the body. Such an approach to exercise provides you with the most effective, time-efficient program possible. Later in this book you'll find detailed step-by-step instructions for designing your own personal exercise program, custom-tailored to your particular goals.

Myth #3:
"Different Forms of Exercise Use Different Muscles"

Some people believe that "running uses different muscles than swimming does, and a weight lifting session uses still different muscles." Actually, these types of exercise in general involve the same set of muscles; the difference is in the proportion of the effort extracted from the various individual muscles.

As one small example, consider the leg muscles used when you run as opposed to the leg muscles involved when you swim using the frog kick. It may *seem* as though the frog kick uses the inner and outer thigh muscles, while running calls upon the quadriceps (the large muscles along the front of the thighs).

In fact, both exercises use *all* of the leg muscles. Running does extract a higher percentage of the effort from the quadriceps, but rest assured that the inner and outer thigh muscles are also working when you run. Likewise, your quadriceps do participate in the frog kick, even though a larger portion of the work is done by the inner and outer thigh muscles.

A more meaningful way to categorize exercise is to identify whether the activity is aerobic or anaerobic in nature. The factor which determines a given exercise's category is not which muscles are used or even which motion is involved. The critical factor is how the required energy is produced, via an anaerobic pathway or an aerobic pathway. And the factors determining which energy pathway is used are the duration of the activity and its intensity.

Immediate and short-term energy is produced in the muscles by means of chemical processes which do not require oxygen and are thus called anaerobic. (The word "anaerobic" means "in the absence of oxygen.")

If the exertion continues beyond about a minute and a half, depending on its intensity, the aerobic pathways are called upon to supply the required energy. These pathways are called aerobic because they *do* require air; (the word "aerobic" means "in the presence of oxygen.")

Aerobic exercise, then, is activity which activates and strengthens the aerobic energy pathways by enhancing the cardiorespiratory system's ability to get oxygen to the stressed area quickly enough and in sufficient quantities to sustain the activity, while anaerobic exercise is activity which activates and strengthens the anaerobic energy pathways by enhancing the muscles' ability to produce energy without oxygen on an immediate or short-term basis.

In more readily identifiable terms, aerobic exercise is activity which intensifies your breathing and elevates your heart rate. To be effective, aerobic exercise must be performed at the proper pace and for a period of time. Although the aerobic energy pathways "kick in" after about a minute and a half, it has been determined that a minimum of 12 minutes is required for aerobic exercise to produce any training effect. The proper pace is most easily determined by your heart rate. In Section 4, I'll describe how to determine your personal aerobic heart rate.

Aerobic exercise strengthens your cardiorespiratory system. It's also the best method around for eliminating unwanted fat from your body while improving muscle tone, a process I call "de-massing." (More on this point shortly.) Section 5 describes the aerobic exercises I've designed for de-massing. When de-massing is not your goal and you seek only to strengthen your cardiorespiratory system, you can use other forms of aerobic exercise as discussed in Section 4.

Anaerobic exercise generally involves repeated short bursts of intense effort which momentarily push your heart rate above the aerobic level. In response, muscles become larger and stronger, which is generally the goal.

Weight lifting is the most common form of this type of anaerobic exercise because it's the most effective at achieving this goal. Section 6 describes the most efficient weight lifting exercises I've found.

In addition, there's a second type of anaerobic exercise: activity which stresses the muscles but does not raise your heart rate to the aerobic level. Such exercises are generally used to maintain muscle size and strength or as at-home substitutes for weight routines. See Section 7.

Myth #4:
"Spot Reducing Can Remove Fat Selectively"

This myth has some appearance of logic to it. If you want to get rid of a particular bulge of fat, doesn't it stand to reason that exercising that area would burn it off? Or that you could attack it from the outside and vibrate or steam it off?

The truth is that external approaches simply don't work. Vibrating or jiggling fat doesn't make it go away. Devices like sweat suits, saunas, or inflated belts or pants cause you to lose body fluids in the form of sweat, not burned fat. And, because the smaller muscle groups lose fluids more readily than do the larger muscle groups, you probably won't lose fluids from the areas you might expect with such devices. (Ever notice how your face is the first part of your body to become flushed in a sauna?) The real point, however, is that any losses you do achieve will be strictly temporary. As soon as the lost fluids are replaced, any reduced areas resume their original sizes.

Exercise *is* the answer, if properly done, but the cause and effect relationship is not direct from the exercised muscles to the subcutaneous fat (fat beneath the skin) in that area.

Fat accumulates in areas not exercised properly. It is withdrawn from storage only when caloric demands dictate, and is generally withdrawn on a last-in-first-out basis. That is, when fat is needed for fuel, it is generally removed first from wherever it was most recently deposited, then from the area in which it was next most recently deposited, and so on. Fat is removed from the area being exercised only by coincidence.

How, then, is exercise the answer? In three ways. First, proper exercise helps create the caloric demand necessary to initiate fat withdrawal. Second, exercising a given muscle properly *can* eliminate intramuscular fat

(fat within the muscle tissue). When intramuscular fat is removed, the muscle loses its out-of-shape shape (short and thick) and adopts its in-shape shape (long and thin), and it is the shape of the muscles over the bone structure which gives a body its shape. And third, proper exercise stimulates the production of the enzymes which break down fat, that's why just losing weight doesn't give you back your youthful shape. Weight loss alone eliminates only subcutaneous fat, leaving the muscles short and thick and you with the same shape, only smaller.*

To eliminate intramuscular fat, you exercise the muscles aerobically– i.e., with your heart rate elevated to the proper level for a continuous period of time. Otherwise, exercise will cause the muscles to increase in size, precisely what you *don't* want if you're trying to reduce the area. (More on performing aerobic exercises properly in Sections 4 and 5.)

Myth #5:
"Carbohydrates Are Fattening"

A traditional way to "go on a diet" has long been to cut out all those "fattening" carbohydrates: potatoes, pasta, bread, and the like. Such a strategy indeed lowers total calorie intake, but only if you don't replace the omitted items with calories in other forms.

There are at least two problems with this method, however. First, people cutting down on carbohydrates all too often increase their consumption of proteins and fats. The problem here is (to put it simply) that fats are bad for you. Second, some of those "fattening" carbohydrates are (again, to put it simply) the very best types of foods around for building a sound mind and healthy body. More on this subject in Section 3.

Myth #6:
"Your Weight Is The Truest Measure of Your Progress"

The scale is designed to indicate the total amount of weight placed on it. It cannot take into account the distribution of that weight, and that distribution is the key to your appearance.

The mirror, in fact, is the truest indicator of what shape your body is in. By accurately reflecting your height and weight ratio, it shows all the good points ... and the precise locations of any problem areas.

One final thing to remember: Muscle outweighs fat by about 2 to 1. If you remove fat from your body and improve muscle tone at the same time, you may actually see a net *gain* in weight registered on your scale, but your mirror will show a stronger, trimmer, and more attractive you.

Myth #7:
"Women Become Overly Muscular If They Lift Weights"

Because a woman's musculature is far less dense than a man's, it's anatomically impossible for a woman to reach the state of muscular development seen in some men. Women should feel free to use weights to attain their body contouring goals.

(Note to anyone afraid of becoming "muscle-bound" if they lift weights: If your mirror shows any muscles developing beyond where you want them, simply adjust your program accordingly. More on this in Section 4.)

Myth #8:
"Some Older People Stay Overweight No Matter What They Do"

This line of thinking goes something like this: No matter how much or what kind of exercise some older people get, they will become and stay overweight, that for this type of person, being overweight is an inevitable part of the aging process.

In reality, nothing could be further from the truth.

It *is* true that many people become (and remain) overweight as they get older, but their excess weight is *not* due to some unavoidable trick of "fate." What actually happens is quite simple. As some people get older, they tend gradually to grow away from the physically demanding activities of their younger years but don't change their eating habits. The inevitability here should be obvious: the same caloric intake with less calories burned equals *fat*!

The basic solution should be obvious, too: changes in eating habits and/or stepped-up activity levels. The specific solution for a given individual is to finish reading this book and design a fitness program that meets his or her own particular needs, remembering that the best way to eliminate existing fat is with proper exercise.

Myth #9:
"But I Don't Have Time To Exercise!"

Actually, this may be the number 1 misconception there is about fitness: that vast amounts of time are required to get and stay fit. If your fitness program is properly designed, it will give you the results you seek in the minimum time possible because it will be focused precisely and exclusively on *your* objectives.

And where will you find such a program? Read on ...

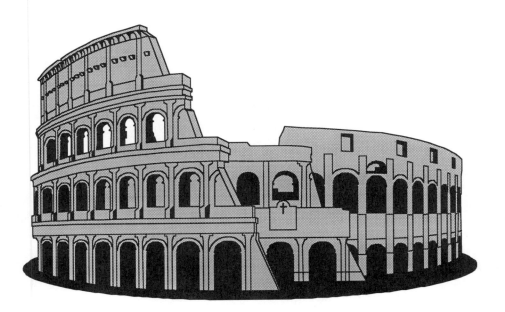

---

*   Except in extreme cases when ALL subcutaneous fat has been removed and muscle tissue must be burned for fuel.

Chapter 2: Getting Started

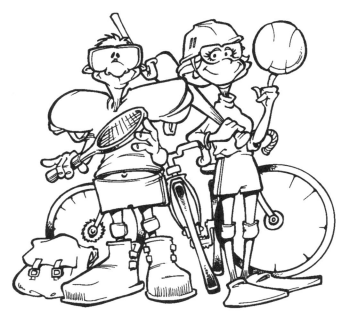

Before you can start your new fitness program, you need to design that program.

Before you can design your program, you need to define the specific goals you intend to achieve with it.

Before you can define those goals, you need to locate your personal starting point.

Now we can get started.

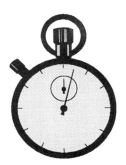

Where Are You Now?

First, assess the current condition of your body, in terms of both how it looks and how it functions.

Evaluate How Your Body Currently Operates

If you're over 30 and/or have a history of heart problems, consult your doctor before launching any new fitness program. A treadmill stress test is the very best way of assessing your heart's condition.

Assuming that your doctor gives you his or her blessing, think about how a fitness program could *improve* the way your body functions. Would you like to lower your heart rate? Increase your stamina? Wish you had stronger arms, stronger legs?

Make a list of all these improvements, stating them as goals with specific objectives. For example, you might say: "I'd like to be able to climb those stairs without getting out of breath." Or, you might say: "My hang gliding instructor assures me that no great amount of strength is required once I get airborne, but suggests that a 110-pound woman like me will have an easier time handling the equipment on the ground if I build up my arm strength." Or, you might say: "My doctor recommends lowering my resting heart rate by 10 beats a minute."

Define high goals for yourself, but don't set yourself up for failure. Be sure that all your goals are realistically attainable with a fitness program. Even the most effective fitness program imaginable can't make you taller, change your basic bone structure, or give you smaller ears. (You may be amazed, however, at the changes you *can* make.)

Evaluate Your Body's Current Appearance

This step may be a toughie, but it's vital to the success of your program. Strip down and look–really ***look***–at yourself in a mirror from every angle.

Remember, the mirror is the truest indicator of what shape your body is in and unequivocally (sometimes unmercifully) reveals any problem areas. (If you're dismayed by what the mirror shows you, cheer up: that same mirror will provide proof positive of the results of an effective fitness program like the one you'll be designing. You may dread looking at your body now, but you'll come to regard the mirror as a friend.)

Congratulate yourself on the things that please you about what you see. Then take careful note of any and all areas you wish you could change. Take your time about this, and do lots of "if only–fantasizing: "I wouldn't look too bad if only ..." or better: "I'd look terrific if only ..." be specific: "I like the way my legs are shaped, basically. If only I didn't have that ugly cellulite at the top of my thighs ..." or: "My upper body's in pretty good shape; if only I could beef up those skinny legs ..."

Again, limit your "wish list" to things realistically within your power to modify. While remarkable results are certainly possible with a good fitness program, there are *some* limits.

Where Are You Going From Here?

What would it take to make your fantasies about the way your body looks and functions come true? A few inches off here, a few added there? A stronger heart, stronger lungs?

Make a list of your goals, stating them in specific terms: "Eliminate cellulite from outer thighs and backs of legs;" "Increase arm strength;" "Flatten stomach;" "Eliminate 'love handles';" "Firm up upper arms;" "Increase stamina;" "Take two inches off waist;" etc.

How Are You Going To Get There?

Now that you've defined where you are currently, envisioned where you want to be, and determined the specific goals you need to attain in order to get there, how are you going to achieve those goals?

Simple. You're going to design your very own exercise program. You're going to follow through with that program. You're also going to learn what foods you should be eating and which you should avoid and you're going to make appropriate adjustments to your eating habits.

Chapter 3: About Your Eating Habits ...

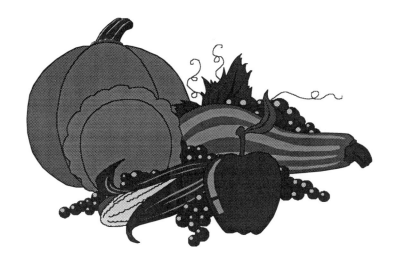

OK, I admit it. The real reason we exercise properly is to earn the right to eat again.

Seriously, eating *is* a real pleasure, but *what* you eat makes a tremendous difference. It can complement all that exercise and contribute to your health and well-being ... or it can undermine all your good efforts.

As I said in the beginning of this book, I don't expect you to suddenly begin following all my suggestions to the letter. I can only encourage you to follow them whenever you can and to gradually make them a part of your everyday patterns.

The phrase "as often as possible" appears several times throughout this discussion. Bear in mind, however, that the more often you find it possible to heed the guidelines, the faster you'll feel and see results.

Two Simple Rules

There are just two basic rules, really:

- Complex carbohydrates are the best kinds of food you can consume; eat them as often as you want.

- Fats are harmful; avoid them as often as possible.

The reasons behind these rules have been stated in more detail–and more emphatically–elsewhere by many nutritional experts, most notably Nathan Pritikin. (See The Pritikin Program for Diet & Exercise by Nathan Pritikin and Patrick M. McGrady, Jr., published by Grosset & Dunlap.)

Why Complex Carbohydrates Are Encouraged

Complex carbohydrates–grains, most vegetables, fruits, pasta, rice–are simply the most beneficial types of food for human beings:

- Fibers from skin pulp helps to scrub away cling fats throughout the body.

- They are the most efficiently metabolized.

- They are the best sources of vitamins, minerals, energy, and fiber.

- They provide a stable supply of glucose, the brain's only fuel.

Why Fats Are To Be Avoided

Fatty foods–most meats, some fish, nuts, oily vegetables such as avocados, dairy products, and oils–should be avoided because their consumption all too quickly translates into an excessive level of fat in the bloodstream, and excess fat in the bloodstream is harmful to your body in at least four ways:

- They are not water soluble like carbohydrates and protein groups.

- It interferes with carbohydrate metabolism and encourages diabetes.

- It causes a rise in cholesterol and uric levels in the tissues, contributing to arteriosclerosis (hardening of the arteries) and gout.

- It causes elements of the blood to stick together and clog small blood vessels and capillaries, depriving tissues of oxygen and thereby impairing peak mental and physical performance.

Since nearly all foods contain some amount of fat, you run virtually no risk of consuming too little fat if you avoid fatty foods. The danger lies at the other end of the scale, in consuming too much. Fat intake should not exceed more than 30% of energy content of the diet, at least 50% should be unsaturated fats.

A Few Other Things To Avoid

You can further improve the quality of your diet by avoiding as often as possible:

- High-cholesterol foods such as egg yolks, shrimp, caviar, and organ meats. (Always knew there was a good reason I shouldn't eat liver!)

- All forms of processed sugar. Processed sugar is too concentrated for the body to deal with efficiently. One candy bar introduces as much sugar into your system as *five* apples or oranges eaten at one sitting.

- All forms of caffeine and alcohol. Both substances interfere with proper digestion.

- Salt added during cooking or while eating.

- All soft drinks, including the diet varieties. Carbon dioxide (CO_2) in such a concentrated form increases the level of carbon (a chemical bonding agent) in the bloodstream, reducing the amount of hydrogen used by oxygen in the electronic transport process to form water (i.e., "sweat"), especially during exercise.

What About Proteins?

The human body requires a certain amount of protein for repairing, replacing, and protecting tissues against becoming over stressed. (Endorphin peptides are secreted in the brain, and have a pain relieving effect like morphine.) Peptides are compounds formed from two or more amino acids linkage with carboxyl group or by the hydrolysis of proteins.

Too much protein (more than about 16% of your total calories) causes your body to lose many important minerals. Excess protein also creates toxins in the blood. These toxins, if combined with insufficient glucose resulting from insufficient carbohydrate intake, can result in hypoglycemia (an abnormal drop in blood sugar). Symptoms of hypoglycemia are weakness, light-headedness, and fatigue.

Another problem with protein consumption is that many of the traditional sources of protein are also high in undesirable elements: fats (as in most meats, milk, cheeses, and other dairy products) or cholesterol (as in eggs, shrimp, and organ meats).

As often as possible, eat low-fat forms of protein: white meat of poultry, non-fatty fish, or vegetable sources such as grains, tubers, and iron-rich garden variety beans. Limit your protein consumption to around 16% of your total caloric consumption. Remember that complex carbohydrates provide calcium and proteins (try some dark green leafy vegetables or some legumes); you don't have to eat meat, eggs, milk, or cheese to get your daily protein.

Recommended daily protein intake is about 0.9g per Kg body weight. (To determine your daily protein requirement in grams, multiply your weight in pounds by 0.424.) This recommendation holds even for people who are under or overweight.

To help the conversion process, remember 1 Kg = 1000 grams = 35.3 oz. = 2.2 lbs.

Vitamins and Minerals

You're probably already aware that adequate quantities of vitamins and minerals are essential for efficient muscle movement and development as well as for optimal health. Did you also know that nearly all these requirements can be met with complex carbohydrates? Grains offer folacin, niacin, B-1, B-6, K, magnesium, and iron; legumes offer folacin, niacin, biotin, choline, B-2, calcium, magnesium, and iron; vegetables offer folacin, biotin, choline, A, B-6, E, iodine, calcium, magnesium, and iron; fruits offer K and potassium; citrus fruits, tomatoes, green peppers, and salad greens offer C. You don't *have* to consume dairy products to get calcium (try some dark green leafy vegetables or some legumes), and you don't *have* to consume meat to get B vitamins (try some vegetables or grains).

The carrot, apple and celery combination provides every mineral known to the human race.

Only vitamins B-12 and D are not available in some form of plant food. Nonfat milk can provide both, and lean meat offers vitamin B-12, or use liquid, powder, or tablet supplements for these vitamins and any other vitamins or minerals you suspect may not be provided in sufficient quantities by the foods you normally eat.

Along with making sure that you consume *enough* vitamins and minerals, take care that you don't consume *too much*. Just as vitamin and mineral deficiencies can cause disease and other problems (e.g., scurvy from insufficient vitamin C, rickets from insufficient calcium), excessive levels of some vitamins (niacin, A, C, D, E, and K) and any mineral can have negative effects.

For example, insufficient iron can lead to iron-deficiency anemia, but an excess of iron can cause siderosis and cirrhosis of the liver; an iodine deficiency can cause goiter (enlarged thyroid), but too much iodine can depress thyroid activity which can in turn slow the cells' resting metabolic level. Besides, I've never seen any documented proof that you can enhance exercise performance with vitamin/mineral supplements beyond the U.S. Food and Drug Administration's Recommended Daily Allowances.

For more details on vitamins and minerals, see Chapter 2 of Exercise Physiology by William D. McArdle, Frank I. Katch, and Victor L. Katch, published by Lea & Febiger, or any other authoritative source.

A Few More "Do's" and "Don'ts"

The following are not rules, exactly–they're more like tips that can contribute to sound eating habits.

- Listen to that voice from your childhood and *eat slowly*. Put your fork down between bites and chew your food thoroughly.

- Eat food fresh whenever possible and in as close to its natural state as possible. Don't overcook foods and avoid processed foods.

- Don't fast. This one *is* a rule. Recall that glucose is the brain's only source of fuel, and the body can store only very limited quantities of glucose.

- Time your eating to get the most out of it. Eating a number of small meals throughout the day is the most productive method of consuming food. Consuming one meal a day, large or small, is nearly as unproductive as fasting.

- If you find yourself in a social situation faced with "to be avoided" items, eat portions of everything out of politeness to your host or hostess, but make those portions small out of consideration for the health and good looks of your best friend - you!

- When you order a pasta dish in a restaurant, ask to have the sauce served separately. (Sauces are typically high in fat content, and most chefs are overly generous with the sauce. Besides, pasta has an enjoyable flavor of its own.) Ditto for dressings on salads.

- Miss Manners, where are you when I need you most? Regardless of what the etiquette books may say, requesting sauces and dressings on the side has become second nature to me.

- If you develop an intense craving for one of those foods you're trying to avoid, allow yourself a *small* portion. In many cases, a small portion will satisfy the craving.

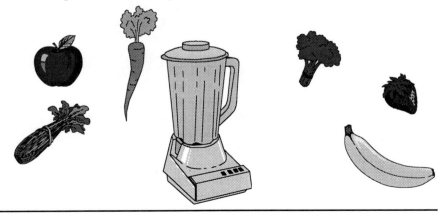

Ireland's Edge Blend

Athletes or working executives on tight schedules can conveniently create a vitamin, mineral and complex carbohydrate rich smoothie by using a food blender. Start by pouring 2 1/2 cups of fruit juice and add a 1/2 apple, one celery stalk, one carrot stick, 4 strawberries, handful of spinach, two potato slices and one whole banana, which is an absolute drink must to insure smoothie texture and desirable fruit taste. You can drink this smoothie blend before, during, or after an activity. It takes 5 minutes to make and can be poured into a sports bottle.

- Drinking enough water benefits weight lost by eliminating body dehydration that causes fluid retention forming extra weight in puffy and swollen tissues. Experts recommend drinking up to 20 ounces (2 1/2 cups) of water in an hour or two preceding exercise, and drinking 3-6 oz. (1/2 cup) every 10-20 minutes during the exercise session. Remember cool water enters the digestive tract faster than warm liquids.

- To prevent the dehydration process, consume fluids before the body becomes thirsty.

- When performing a 90 minute plus activity at a 75% maximum heart rate level requires sugar, potassium and electrolyte replacement. A three-part water and one-part apple juice diluted mixture would be a good replacement source.

- The prudent diets should contain at least 60% to 70% of its calories in the form of carbohydrates, predominantly starches.

- A calorie is a unit of heat used to express the energy value of food. As a general rule foods that are high in water are low in calories. The total daily energy requirement is about 2100 and 2700 calories for women and men, respectively. For the endurance athletes, the daily food intake should supply about 4000 calories. Burning 250 calories a day and reducing calorie intake by 250 calories a day will add up to approximately a 1 pound loss each week.

- Please refer to the exercise calorie chart to aid yourself in figuring out how many calories your exercise activity burns per minute according to your body weight.

Exercise Calorie Chart

Activity	Calories Burned per min. by weight				
Body Weight	110	130	150	170	190
Badminton	4.9	5.7	6.6	7.5	8.3
Basketball	6.9	8.1	9.4	10.6	11.9
Canoeing, leisure	2.2	2.6	3.0	3.4	3.8
Canoeing, racing	5.2	6.1	7.0	7.0	8.9
Card Playing	1.3	1.5	1.7	1.9	2.2
Cleaning	3.1	3.7	4.2	4.8	5.3
Cycling, leisure (9.5 mph)	5.0	5.0	6.8	7.7	8.6
Cycling, racing	8.5	10.0	11.5	13.0	14.5
Dancing, ballroom	2.6	3.0	3.5	3.9	4.4
Dancing, disco	5.2	6.1	7.0	7.9	8.9
Eating, sitting	1.2	1.4	1.6	1.8	2.0
Golf	4.3	5.0	5.8	6.5	7.3
Gymnastics	3.3	3.9	4.5	5.1	5.7
Hiking, no load	6.1	7.1	8.2	9.4	10.3
Hiking, 22# load	7.0	8.3	9.5	10.8	12.0
Horseback riding, walking	2.1	2.4	2.8	3.2	3.5
Horseback riding, galloping	6.9	8.1	9.3	10.6	11.8
Judo	9.8	11.5	13.3	15.0	16.8
Mopping floors	3.1	3.7	4.2	4.8	5.3
Par Course/Circuit Training	9.3	10.9	12.6	14.2	15.9
Racquetball	7.4	8.5	10.0	12.1	14.8
Running, cross country	8.2	9.6	11.1	12.6	14.0
Running, horiz: 11.5 min/mile	6.8	8.0	9.2	10.5	11.7
Running, horiz: 9.5 min/mile	9.7	11.4	13.1	14.9	16.6
Running, horiz: 8.5 min/mile	10.8	12.5	14.2	16.0	17.7
Running, horiz: 7.5 min/mile	12.2	13.9	15.6	17.4	19.1
Running, horiz: 6.5 min/mile	13.9	15.6	17.3	19.1	20.8
Skating, roller and ice	4.7	5.3	6.0	7.0	8.4
Sitting	1.1	1.2	1.4	1.6	1.8
Skiing, level w/hard snow	7.2	8.4	9.7	11.0	12.3
Skiing, moderate speed	6.0	7.0	8.1	9.2	10.2
Skiing, uphill or max speed	13.7	16.2	18.6	21.1	23.6
Skiing, soft snow–leisure	4.9	5.8	6.7	7.5	8.4
Squash, Paddle Tennis	10.6	12.5	14.4	16.3	18.2
Swimming, backstroke	8.5	10.0	11.5	13.0	14.5
Swimming, breast stroke	8.1	9.6	11.0	12.5	13.9
Swimming, fast crawl	7.8	9.2	10.6	12.0	13.4
Swimming, slow crawl	6.4	7.6	8.7	9.9	11.0
Swimming, slow treading	3.1	3.7	4.2	4.8	5.3
Swimming, fast treading	8.5	10.0	11.6	13.1	14.6
Table Tennis	3.4	4.0	4.6	5.2	5.8
Tennis	5.5	6.4	7.4	8.4	9.4
Volleyball	2.5	3.0	3.4	3.9	4.3
Walking, normal pace on ashpalt	4.1	4.7	5.4	6.2	6.9
Walking, normal pace off road	4.6	4.8	5.6	6.3	7.1
Weight Training, free weights	4.3	5.1	5.9	6.7	7.5
Weight Training, weight mach.	6.4	7.6	8.8	10.0	11.2
Weight Training, hydraulic mach.	6.5	7.7	8.9	10.1	11.3

Getting It Together: Eating Habits

- If small portions of "forbidden" foods don't do the job and you decide to break the rules in a big way–that you simply must have that juicy 16-ounce steak, that double-decker bacon cheeseburger, or that triple-dip hot fudge sundae–go ahead, but remember...

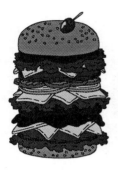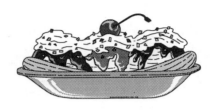

Ireland's Rule For Intelligent Cheating

Never consume nonproductive foods prior to or during a physically demanding activity; consume them after the event if you must consume them at all.

If your system is trying to digest one of these "forbidden" foods (a taxing process under the best of circumstances) at the same time you're trying to partake in a physically demanding activity, your performance of that activity will suffer. On the other hand, your performance will also suffer on an empty stomach. Try to keep your stomach busy with something that's easy for it to work on and which will also supply energy, such as a vegetable or starch of some form.

If the craving for that "forbidden food" simply won't go away, bribe yourself with the promise that you can have it *after* the event.

Don't wallow in guilt if you do "go off the wagon." I'm a firm believer that occasional breaks are a necessary part of any eating "regimen." Is it realistic to say that you'll *never* have a hot fudge sundae again? Is it reasonable to believe you're a bad person, a hopeless failure, if you do? Isn't it possible that you could earn the right to that hot fudge sundae?

Chapter 4: Your Exercise Program; The Schedule

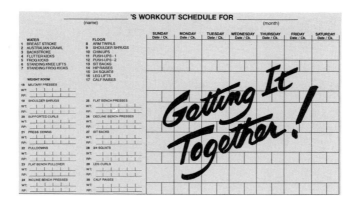

You've assessed the current state of your body, defined the specific things you want to change about it, acknowledged why your current fitness program (or lack of one) hasn't produced the results you want, and vowed to start eating healthy by avoiding fats and eating lots of complex carbohydrates.

There's still one other major component of your overall plan to be put into place, and that's your exercise program.

Designing your own personal exercise program involves three steps. Begin by selecting the individual exercises that will let you most efficiently achieve your particular goals. Then assemble those exercises into a workout schedule. Lastly, follow that schedule and *do* the exercises! As you follow through with your new program, keep a close watch on your progress, as reflected by your mirror, *not* by your scale.

In other words, take the following steps to develop an exercise program to accomplish your specific fitness goals.

As an aid to monitoring your progress, take a picture of yourself in your bathing suit at this point. Your mental self-image will probably lag behind reality as you follow through with your program, and you may become discouraged because you don't *feel* like you're getting anywhere when you are. A "before" picture to compare with the current you in your mirror provides concrete proof of your progress ... an incentive to continue with your program.

Step 1: Select Specific Exercises

The following sections of this book provide detailed instructions on several exercises, arranged according to their primary purposes:

- For "De-Massing," Strengthening Cardiorespiratory System–Use these exercises to eliminate unwanted fat while improving muscle tone ("de-massing") and/or to strengthen your cardiorespiratory system.

- For Building and Strengthening Muscles–Use these exercises for increasing the size and strength of selected muscles.

- For Maintenance–Use these exercises once you've achieved your goals (or as "at-home" substitutes for your other exercises).

- Use the following lists to choose the specific individual exercise(s) best suited to reaching each goal on your list.

Tip:
Most athletic activities require stamina from the lower body, which you can build with aerobic exercise, and/or strength from the upper body, which you develop with anaerobic exercise.

For De-Massing	For Exercise:	Page(s):
shoulders	arms-only water routine	86-90
arms	arms-only water routine	86-90
back	arms-only water routine	86-90
chest	arms-only water routine	86-90

waist	legs-only water routine	92-98
stomach	legs-only water routine	92-98
buttocks	legs-only water routine	92-98
thighs	legs-only water routine	92-98
calves	legs-only water routine	92-98

For Strengthening/Maintaining Cardiorespiratory System:

If you have selected any of the exercises listed above and perform them correctly, they will provide sufficient aerobic exercise to strengthen your cardiorespiratory system. If your list of objectives does not include any "trim it down, tone it up" (i.e., de-massing) goals, you'll need to add some form of aerobics to your list of exercises. More on this topic shortly.

For Building/Strengthening	See Exercise:	Page:
chest & arms	pullover	61
neck	shoulder shrugs	65
shoulders	military presses	63
shoulders	shoulder shrugs	65
chest	pullover	61
arms	supported curls	67
arms	press downs	69
chest	flat bench presses	75
back	pull downs	71
chest & arms	pullover	61
chest:	bench presses:	
upper	incline	73
middle	flat	75
lower	decline	77
stomach	sit backs	79
thighs	3/4 squats	81
(hamstrings)	leg curls	83
buttocks	3/4 squats	81
buttocks	leg curls	83
calves	calf raises	85

Getting It Together: Your Exercise Program

For Maintaining:	See Exercise:	Page:
necks	shoulder shrugs	124
shoulders	arm twirls	123
shoulders	shoulder shrugs	124
shoulders	chin ups	125
arms	chin ups	125
arms	push ups - 1	127
arms	push ups - 2	128
chest	push ups - 1	127
chest	push ups - 2	128
stomach	sit backs	130
buttocks	hip raises	131
buttocks	3/4 squats	132
thighs	3/4 squats	132
thighs	leg lifts	134
calves	calf raises	135

Note

If you're an athlete training for a particular event, you'll need to continue performing the activities related to that event as a key element of your program. That is, if you're training to be a sprinter, you'll need to keep running sprints. Use the exercises described in this book to augment, but not replace, your event-specific training.

Step 2: Devise Your Workout Schedule

After making your selections, organize the individual exercises into a schedule of daily routines.

List "Your" Exercises On Separate Sheets of Paper

As you review your list of goals, you may find that some exercises appear next to more than one goal, or that you have noted more than one exercise next to some goals. Organize your goal/exercise information by writing each exercise you've selected on a separate piece of paper, along with the goal or goals it addresses.

Categorize the Exercises

Now sort the exercises into categories, heeding the following guidelines.

Separate Upper Body Exercises From Lower Body Exercises

First, divide your exercises into two categories: those involving the upper body and those involving the lower body. You'll get results more quickly if you don't work both areas of your body on the same day.

Here's why: When you exercise, blood rushes to the area to supply the chemical processes initiated by the stress to the muscles. (These processes continue long after the activity stops, commonly into the following day.) If the next area you exercise is adjacent to or near the first (e.g., stomach then chest), your body can maintain sufficient blood supplies to both areas. If, however, the second area is far removed from the first (e.g., shoulders then thighs), your body is forced to withdraw some of the blood supply from the first area in order to supply the second, interrupting the transformation processes you worked so hard to initiate in the first.

Trying to exercise both areas on the same day thus hinders maximum results because the first area doesn't get the full benefits of the exercise. Plan to work on either the upper body *or* the lower body on a given day, but not both.

Separate De-Massing Exercises From Building Exercises

De-massing and building require different bodily states. Therefore, if either of your two categories (upper body and lower body) include some exercises for building and others for de-massing, subdivide the categories accordingly. Exercises for strengthening your cardiorespiratory system can go in either the "de-mass upper body" category or the "de-mass lower body" category.

Assign Exercises To Specific Days

At this point, you have as many as four categories of exercises: "de-mass upper body," "de-mass lower body," "build upper body," and "build lower body." (There's no requirement, of course, that you have all four categories. If it is not your goal to build your lower body, for example, you don't have a "build lower" category.) These categories represent the basic guideline for assigning exercises to specific days on your schedule: on a given day, exercise just one section of your body (upper or lower), and work on either de-massing or building that section. Do not mix categories on the same day.

If your goals call for both de-massing and building a section of your body, you'll reach both goals most efficiently if you start with a "de-mass only" program for that section and postpone the building exercises until you've eliminated all unwanted fat from that section. Once you've achieved your de-massing goals, you can switch to de-mass maintenance routines for that section and add routines for building and strengthening. Maintenance exercises can be mixed with other categories on a given day.

You can now begin assigning categories of exercises to specific slots on your schedule using one of the log sheets provided at the end of this book. I recommend that you *not* exercise every day. Working out five or six days a week provides sufficient exercise to effect the changes you seek and gives your body one or two days "off" to rebuild, and gives you one or two days to celebrate your new look and feel.

How you schedule those days within each week depends entirely on what best fits with your other activities. (Personally, I prefer to work out on week days and take weekends off.) It's not important how your schedule is structured. It *is* important that you have a schedule. Unless exercising becomes a normal, planned part of your routine, it's entirely too easy to find that you "just don't have time."

As you assign exercises to specific days, keep the following points in mind.

Include Sufficient Aerobic Exercise In Your Schedule

Because aerobic exercise is so crucial to getting and staying fit, your schedule should include some sessions calling for at least 12 minutes of continuous activity with your heart rate elevated to its effective aerobic level. (I'll describe how to calculate your proper heart rate later in this section.)

If your program involves exercises aimed at de-massing target areas, this requirement is easily met since de-massing requires that the exercises be performed aerobically. Just be sure that in performing the exercises, your heart rate remains elevated to the proper level and you don't stop for a break for at least 12 minutes. (I'll also discuss how to monitor your heart rate later in this section.)

If your program currently includes only exercises for building target areas, you'll need to add some aerobic exercise to your schedule. As I explained in Section 1, I don't recommend any of the traditional forms (running, jogging, skipping rope, aerobic dancing, jumping jacks, and the like).

Fortunately, there are a number of positive ways to add aerobic exercise to a "build-it-up"-only program:

Recommended outdoor aerobics:

- Vigorous walking
- Bicycling
- Cross–country skiing
- Roller skating
- Ice skating

Recommended indoor aerobics:

- Chair stepping
- Treadmill machine
- Rowing machine
- Trampoline
- Floor exercises that do not conflict with the rest of your workout; see Chapter 7.

Swimming, either outdoors or inside, is an excellent way to get aerobic exercise when your program otherwise includes no aerobic work.

Follow Recommended Session Minimums and Maximums

In mapping out a given day's routine, follow the recommended minimums and maximums specified in the exercise descriptions in the following sections. Please don't ignore the recommended maximums in an effort to hasten results. Your muscles can maintain the optimum state for exercise only for the stated times; attempting to exercise beyond those limits inevitably overstresses the muscles and is thus counterproductive.

Further, overdoing during an exercise session can adversely affect your health by wearing down your body's immunities. Lastly, overdoing is no fun. If it's no fun, you'll probably dread it after a while, and if you come to dread it, you'll probably find some reason to give it up.

Order Exercises According to Muscle Sizes Involved

In a given session, work the large muscle groups first and then the small muscle groups. (The large muscles of the upper body are the chest, shoulder, and back muscles; the small muscles of the upper body are the arm, face, and neck muscles. In the lower body, the large muscles are the buttock and thigh muscles; small lower body muscles are the stomach, hamstring, and calf muscles.) Remember, the large muscle groups can withstand far more exertion before altering their resting states than the small muscle groups can. If you exert the small muscles first, they won't be able to fully support the larger muscles when it's their turn.

Allow Time In Each Session For Stretching

A few minutes of stretching, preferably before *and* after your workout, can enhance the exercise and increase your flexibility. Before a workout, stretching acts to get the muscles warmed up, relaxed, and ready for action. Stretching after exercising, while your muscles are fully warmed, is an ideal way to increase your flexibility and it's a great way to cool down after a hard workout. One warning: take care when stretching a "cold" muscle. Work up to a full stretch slowly, gently, easily.

Rather than describe specific stretching techniques here, I'll recommend an excellent book on the subject: Stretching, by Robert A. and Jean E. Anderson, published by Shelter Publications, Inc.

Include Time For Enjoying the Post-Workout Glow

If at all possible, avoid having to rush off to your next activity after you work out. Don't jump immediately into the shower. (Getting into a shower without first cooling down can be a shock, potentially even fatal, to your system. Besides, you probably won't feel like jumping anywhere.) Enjoy your favorite cooling-down activity, *then* take a leisurely shower.

Savor the knowledge that the "work" initiated by your workout continues long after you've stopped exercising. Notice how all that pre-workout tension and stress has magically disappeared. Take pleasure in the sensation of being better-equipped than ever to tackle the rest of the day. Look forward to a good night's sleep.

You've earned it–enjoy it!

Devising (and Revising) a Schedule: an Example

Let's consider the case of Fred, a fictitious fellow with a sedentary job, no current fitness program, and a recently-celebrated 40th birthday. Self-assessment seems obligatory at such milestones and Fred finds himself flabby, weak, and without stamina. These general findings translate into an ambitious list of specific goals:

- Eliminate "love handles"
- Flatten stomach
- Take two inches off thighs
- Eliminate flab from upper arms
- Increase stamina
- Increase arm strength
- Firm up chest
- Increase leg strength
- Reduce heart rate by 10 BPM
- Firm up buttocks

First, he selects the exercises that will let him achieve those goals most efficiently and notes them on his list of goals. Fred's list includes some "trim it down" goals (for his stomach, waist, and thighs) and some "firm it up" goals (for his upper arms, chest, and buttocks). Water routines are ideal for these de-massing purposes. And, they'll strengthen his cardiorespiratory system at the same time, thereby increasing his stamina and reducing his heart rate. For increasing his arm and leg strength, Fred selects appropriate weight room exercises.

Fred's list of goals now looks like:

- Eliminate "love handles" - "legs only" water routine
- Flatten stomach - "legs only" water routine
- Take two inches off thighs - "legs only" water routine
- Eliminate flab from upper arms - "arms only" water routine
- Increase stamina - water routines
- Increase arm strength - supported curls, press downs
- Firm up chest - "arms only" water routine
- Increase leg strength - 3/4 squats, leg curls, calf raises
- Reduce heart rate by 10 BPM - water routines
- Firm up buttocks - "legs only" water routine

He then writes each exercise on a separate sheet of paper, noting the goal (or goals) it addresses:

"Legs only" water routine - de-mass stomach, waist, thighs, buttocks; strengthen cardiorespiratory system

"Arms only" water routine - de-mass arms, chest; strengthen cardiorespiratory system

Supported curls - build arm strength

Press downs - build arm strength

3/4 squats - build leg strength

Leg curls - build leg strength

Calf raises - build leg strength

Fred realizes that the most efficient way to proceed is to accomplish his de-massing goals before starting to work with weights. He therefore sets aside the arm- and leg-strengthening exercises for the moment. (If his goals had called for de-massing just the upper body or just the lower body, he could have started his building program for the other section immediately.)

Because he is eager to reach his objectives, Fred decides to work out after work each Monday through Friday and on Saturday mornings. He schedules two hours each day (5 minutes for warm-up stretching, an hour and a half for exercising, and 25 minutes for cool-down stretching, showering, and basking in the glow). He alternates upper body sessions (Monday, Wednesday, and Friday) with lower body sessions (Tuesday, Thursday, and Saturday).

His initial log sheet, then, looks like:

FRED's WORKOUT SCHEDULE FOR **FEB '86**

ACTIVITY		SUNDAY	MONDAY	TUESDAY	WEDNESDAY	THURSDAY	FRIDAY	SATURDAY
WATER ✓1 BREAST STROKE ✓2 AUSTRALIAN CRAWL ✓3 BACKSTROKE 4 FLUTTER KICKS 5 FROG KICKS ✓6 STANDING KNEE LIFTS ✓7 STANDING FROG KICKS OTHER AEROBICS: 8 9	**FLOOR:** 10 ARM TWIRLS 11 SHOULDER SHRUGS 12 CHIN UPS 13 PUSH UPS - 1 14 PUSH UPS - 2 15 SIT BACKS 16 HIP RAISES 17 3/4 SQUATS 18 LEG LIFTS 19 CALF RAISES						⑥⑦	1
WEIGHT ROOM: 20 MILITARY PRESSES wt: rp:	26 FLAT BENCH PRESSES wt: rp:	①②③ 2	⑥⑦ 3	①②③ 4	⑥⑦ 5	①②③ 6	⑥⑦ 7	8
21 SHOULDER SHRUGS wt: rp:	27 DECLINE BENCH PRESSES wt: rp:	①②③ 9	⑥⑦ 10	①②③ 11	⑥⑦ 12	①②③ 13	⑥⑦ 14	15
22 SUPPORTED CURLS wt: rp:	28 SIT BACKS wt: rp:	①②③ 16	⑥⑦ 17	①②③ 18	⑥⑦ 19	①②③ 20	⑥⑦ 21	22
23 PRESS DOWNS wt: rp:	29 3/4 SQUATS wt: rp:	①②③ 23	⑥⑦ 24	①②③ 25	⑥⑦ 26	①②③ 27	28	
24 PULLDOWNS wt: rp:	30 LEG CURLS wt: rp:							
25 INCLINE BENCH PRESSES wt: rp:	31 CALF RAISES wt: rp:							

After a time of diligently following this schedule, Fred sees in his mirror that he's achieved his de-massing goals. It's time to switch to maintenance routines for the de-massed areas and to begin his arm- and leg-strengthening program. His new log sheet looks like:

FRED's WORKOUT SCHEDULE FOR **APRIL '86**

ACTIVITY		SUNDAY	MONDAY	TUESDAY	WEDNESDAY	THURSDAY	FRIDAY	SATURDAY
WATER 1 BREAST STROKE 2 AUSTRALIAN CRAWL 3 BACKSTROKE 4 FLUTTER KICKS 5 FROG KICKS 6 STANDING KNEE LIFTS 7 STANDING FROG KICKS OTHER AEROBICS: 8 9	**FLOOR:** 10 ARM TWIRLS 11 SHOULDER SHRUGS 12 CHIN UPS 13 PUSH UPS - 1 14 PUSH UPS - 2 15 SIT BACKS 16 HIP RAISES 17 3/4 SQUATS 18 LEG LIFTS 19 CALF RAISES			㉒㉓ 1	㉙㉚㉛ 2	①②③ ㉒㉓ 3	⑥⑦ ㉙㉚㉛ 4	
WEIGHT ROOM: 20 MILITARY PRESSES wt: rp:	26 FLAT BENCH PRESSES wt: rp:	①②③ ㉒㉓ 5	⑥⑦ ㉙㉚㉛ 6	㉒㉓ 7	㉙㉚㉛ 8	①②③ ㉒㉓ 9	⑥⑦ ㉙㉚㉛ 10	11
21 SHOULDER SHRUGS wt: rp:	27 DECLINE BENCH PRESSES wt: rp:	①②③ ㉒㉓ 12	⑥⑦ ㉙㉚㉛ 13	㉒㉓ 14	㉙㉚㉛ 15	①②③ ㉒㉓ 16	⑥⑦ ㉙㉚㉛ 17	18
✓22 SUPPORTED CURLS wt: 5,10,15,20,25,15 rp: 10,8,6,4,1,5-10	28 SIT BACKS wt: rp:							
✓23 PRESS DOWNS wt: 5,10,15,20,25,15 rp: 15,11,7,4,1,5-10	✓29 3/4 SQUATS wt: 10,20,30,40,50,30 rp: 10,8,6,4,1,5-10	①②③ ㉒㉓ 19	⑥⑦ ㉙㉚㉛ 20	㉒㉓ 21	㉙㉚㉛ 22	①②③ ㉒㉓ 23	⑥⑦ ㉙㉚㉛ 24	25
24 PULLDOWNS wt: rp:	✓30 LEG CURLS wt: 25,30,35,40,50,30 rp: 10,8,6,4,1,5-10	①②③ ㉒㉓ 26	⑥⑦ ㉙㉚㉛ 27	28	㉒㉓ 29	㉙㉚㉛ 30		
25 INCLINE BENCH PRESSES wt: rp:	✓31 CALF RAISES wt: 10,20,30,40,50,30 rp: 10,8,6,4,1,5-10							

Getting It Together: Your Exercise Program

Step 3: Follow the Program

Once you have your exercise schedule worked out, there is, as they say, "nothing to it but to do it." Keep the following guidelines in mind as you perform the exercises.

Breathe Properly

First of all, remember to breathe! Many people tend to hold their breath while exercising ... and then wonder why they get so tired and light-headed! Beyond that, remember to time your breathing properly. Always inhale just before exerting the body and exhale as you exert it. Exhaling completely is just as important as inhaling fully.

Breathe through your nose rather than through your mouth to filter and warm the air, to prevent drying of your mouth and throat tissues, and to maximize the amount of oxygen available for the oxygen transfer process in the muscles. When you breathe through the mouth, some of the air can escape through the nasal passage before it can be distributed throughout the body via the lungs. Activities involving maximum exertion may require exhaling through both the nose and mouth.

The efficiency of the oxygen transfer process determines how effective the exercise is at producing the changes you seek in the muscles. It also determines how long you can perform the exercise. Efficient oxygen transfer wards off the buildup of lactic acid, which causes muscle fatigue.

When muscle fatigue does occur, the quickest way to regain composure is to concentrate on your breathing as you breathe through your nose. (You can't pant or gasp or hyperventilate through your nose!)

Keep Your Stomach Pulled In

Stomach muscles tend to adopt whatever position they're in during exercise. Thus, if your stomach is pushed out as you exercise, its normal position will tend to become ... pushed out. Unless you have "Develop Stomach Muscles Outward" as one of your goals, keep those muscles pulled in and tight.

Exercise To Proper "Fatigue Level"

Many of the exercise instructions presented in the following sections advise you to continue until the target muscles are "thoroughly fatigued." But just what does that mean?

Well, it means pushing beyond the stage where the muscles are "pretty tired" to the point where they're *really* tired and perhaps beginning to "burn" a bit. *But*: beware of over-fatiguing the muscles. If they begin to quiver and feel incapable of performing their intended functions–if you an barely walk on freshly exercised legs, for example–you've gone too far. Put another way, fatigue is when you can no longer sustain the focused concentration it takes to support the proper breathing technique and the required muscle movements.

Warm Up To Each Exercise

When you begin an exercise, start out slowly and gradually pick up the pace to the appropriate level. (This process usually takes just a few seconds.) Even if you have stretched at the beginning of the workout, the muscles need to be "eased" into each new movement.

Don't Exceed Recommended Maximums

This point was made earlier, but it bears repeating. Don't think you'll get results more quickly by extending the session beyond the recommended maximums. To do so is, at the very least, counterproductive, and at the very worst, hazardous to your health. Overdoing is also a leading cause of "burnouts" disease.

Perform Aerobic Exercises Properly

The idea in aerobic exercise is to get the target area "pumped"–i.e., stressed to the point that blood rushes in–and to continue working the muscles past that point so that the body's stored resources (fat) are called upon. When a muscle is "pumped," it becomes larger, tighter, and firmer to the touch.

To produce the desired aerobic benefits, an exercise must be performed for at least 12 minutes with your heart rate elevated to the proper level. Then move on to the next exercise without stopping for a break.

The entire session should last no longer than an hour and a half since muscles can maintain the "working" state for only about that long. To avoid over stressing the muscles, wearing down your body's immunities, and setting yourself up for burning out, don't extend the session beyond an hour and a half. Stop sooner if the target muscles begin to quiver or you lose your concentration, indicating that the muscles have become overly fatigued.

Determine Your Proper Heart Rate For Aerobic Exercise

The correct level is a percentage of your heart's maximum rate. Since your maximum heart rate is determined primarily by your age, it's easy to calculate: simply subtract your age from 220. When you're 20, your maximum rate is 200 beats per minute; at 30, it's 190, and so on.

The standard percentage of maximum suitable for aerobic exercise is 80%. If your cardiorespiratory system is already in good shape, exercise at 85% of your maximum rate, never higher. If it's in poor shape, start at 75%.

Use the following chart to find the range of heart rates suitable for your age; use the portion of that range appropriate to your current condition.

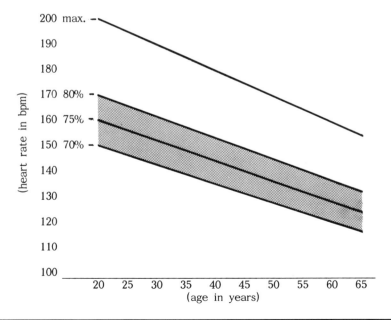

Getting It Together: Your Exercise Program

For example, consider Fred, the fellow we talked about earlier. At 40, he has a maximum heart rate of about 180 beats per minute. Eighty percent of 180 is 144, but since he's starting in relatively poor condition, he chooses (wisely) to begin performing his aerobic workouts at a rate of 136 beats per minute, 75% of his maximum. As his fitness improves he'll be able to increase the rate, but never beyond 85% of maximum, which is 153 beats per minute in his case.

Monitor Your Heart Rate

To determine whether you're exercising at the proper heart rate, monitor your pulse. In the beginning, start the exercise and then pause briefly and count your heart beats at your wrist or jugular vein (in the neck, below the jawbone) for six seconds. Multiply that count by 10 to produce your beats-per-minute rate.

Stop and measure your pulse often and speed up or slow down the exercise according to your readings until you're satisfied that you've reached the appropriate pace. Thereafter, check your pulse only periodically. After a time, checking your pulse at the end of the exercise will be sufficient. Remember, however, that as you get more fit, you'll need to exercise at a faster pace to elevate your heart rate to the proper level.

Use the following heart rate equivalency chart to find the heart rate....number of beats per.

Getting It Together: Your Exercise Program

Heart Rate Equivalency Chart

1 Min	30 Sec	15 Sec	10 Sec
40	20	10	7
45	23	12	8
50	25	13	8
55	28	14	9
60	30	15	10
65	32	16	11
70	35	18	12
75	38	19	13
80	40	20	13
85	43	21	14
90	45	23	15
95	48	24	16
100	50	25	17
105	53	26	18
110	55	28	18
115	58	29	19
120	60	30	20
125	63	31	21
130	65	33	22
135	68	34	23
140	70	35	23
145	73	36	24
150	75	38	25
155	78	39	26
160	80	40	27
165	83	41	28
170	85	43	28
175	88	44	29
180	90	45	30
185	93	46	31
190	95	48	36
195	98	49	33
200	100	50	33
205	103	51	34
210	105	53	35
215	108	54	36
220	110	55	37
225	113	56	38

Getting It Together: Your Exercise Program

For more information on self-monitored aerobic exercise, see Fit or Fat? by Covert Baily, published by the Houghton Mifflin Company.

Remember, the Number One Rule of Exercise

Simply stated, this rule is: if you don't feel it, it isn't working. If you can't feel the muscles in the target area working, you're probably doing the exercise incorrectly. Consult with an instructor before proceeding; unless you can feel it, the exercise isn't serving its intended purpose.

Chapter 5. Water Routines:
Aerobic Exercises For De-Massing; Strengthening Cardiorespiratory System

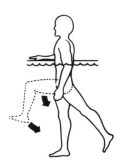

When your goal is to de-mass your body–i.e., to eliminate unwanted fat, including cellulite, while toning your muscles–and/or to strengthen your cardiorespiratory system, the exercise should be aerobic in nature. (Recall that aerobic exercise enhances the cardiorespiratory system's ability to get oxygen to the stressed area quickly enough and in sufficient quantities to support sustained activities.)

This section describes some zero impact full range of motion aerobic exercises I've developed for achieving both these goals. These exercises are all performed in water, for two good reasons.

First, exercising in water is more efficient for these purposes than any other type of exercise, thanks in part to the resistance (10 to 12 lbs.) and support provided by the water. This increased efficiency allows you to achieve your goals more quickly.

Second, when you exercise in water, you don't risk the adverse effects commonly stemming from most gross aerobics: ankle, knee, or back damage, shin splints, and so on. You also avoid the potential damage to joints inherent in such exercises or in working with unsupported weights. In fact, water offers the most therapeutic remedy to these very ailments. Orthopedic surgeons increasingly recommend water activities to their post-surgery outpatients for rehabilitation therapy.

When you exercise outside the water, some of the effort is transferred from the target muscles to the unsupported joints and can lead to overstressing, even damaging, the joints. Water supports your body weight and your joints, allowing the effort to remain focused in the target muscles. If the joints aren't stressed, you don't fatigue as rapidly, and that means you can exercise the muscles longer.

There's an extra bonus. If you participate occasionally in all-out sporting events–that Sunday football game, the twice-a-year squash game with an old buddy, the company picnic softball game–you'll find that the routines in this section are more effective than running, jogging, or other gross aerobics for working out the aches, pains, sore muscles, and bruises that all too often result.

"Well, That All Makes Sense and Sounds Very Fine, But ..."

Did something like this go through your mind as you read the last discussion? Let me see if I can guess how you completed that thought.

"... I Don't Have a Swimming Pool"

You don't have a pool, you say? Is there a YMCA or YWCA in your town? Do you have any friends with pools? Does your town have a community swimming pool? Is there a motel nearby with a swimming pool you might arrange to use? Is there a pool in your local high school? If you look around and exercise a little creative thinking, I bet you'll find that there *is* a pool you can use after all. (The results you'll get will make the effort more than worthwhile.)

Actually, any body of water of sufficient size–a lake, pond, river, ocean, or even a jacuzzi or spa with the temperature lowered to around 80 degrees– can provide a suitable medium as long as you exercise common sense and normal precautions appropriate to that type of water.

Of course, there's always the option of building your very own swimming pool. If space and/or your budget can't accommodate a pool, how about a "swim spa" measuring about 9 by 12 feet for around $7,000? (A swim spa produces a "flow" from one end that allows you to "swim" against it. See your spa dealer for details.)

"... I'm Not a Swimmer" or "... I Can't (or Don't Want to) Get My Head Wet"

Not to worry. None of the routines described in this section require that you be an Olympic-level swimmer. However, you'll probably perform them more efficiently, with less nonproductive motion, if you understand at least basic swimming principles and techniques.

If you don't know how to swim, I recommend that you learn. Low-cost lessons should be available at your local Y, or community pool. Or you can choose from a number of "nonswimmer's" variations of each exercise, ranging from simply holding your head above water to performing the exercise while standing or sitting in water as discussed in the following paragraphs and in the individual exercise descriptions.

How to Perform Water Routines

It's especially important that you take care to avoid exceeding your optimum heart rate for aerobic exercise when using these exercises to de-mass your body and/or strengthen your cardiorespiratory system.

Check your pulse rate frequently until you have determined the pace you need to maintain in order to keep your heart rate at the proper level, less frequently thereafter. Maintain that rate for at least 12 minutes, stopping when the target muscles are thoroughly fatigued. Do not extend the session beyond an hour and a half.

This section describes two types of exercises: those working the upper body and those working the lower body. On a given day, you can combine upper body exercises with other upper body exercises *or* lower body exercises with other lower body exercises. *Don't*, however, do both types on the same day.

The "swimmer's" versions of the exercises involve propelling a buoyant board–a kick board, "boogie" board, or pool buoy–through water, using either just your arms or just your legs. The board should be buoyant enough to support your body easily and should have some "give" to it. The board I use is 24 inches long, 13 inches wide, and 2 inches thick. I'm 6 feet 4 inches tall and weigh 230.

In any version of any of these exercises, a high splash is a sure sign of nonproductive motion, arm stroke or kicking.

For de-massing the upper body ...

To eliminate unwanted fat from your upper body–arms, shoulders, back, chest–develop a routine involving "arms-only" water exercises.

SWIMMERS: Hold the board lightly between your knees and pull yourself through the water using whatever arm motion you prefer: breast stroke, Australian crawl, or backstroke. (Each of these strokes is detailed later in this section.) Hold the board lightly; it's unnecessary and counterproductive to clench your knees firmly.

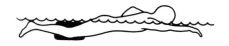

NON-SWIMMERS: The backstroke keeps your face out of the water. Or, you can hold your head above water while performing the breast stroke or Australian crawl. Another option is to perform the exercises while wearing a water jogging device that frees your arms and legs while keeping your head above water. Two such devices are the "Wet Vest," an armless jacket, and "Flugels," inflatable boots and water wings.*

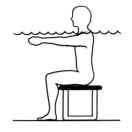

Alternatively, stand or sit in water covering your arms–perhaps even in your bathtub!–and perform the arm motion of your choice. (Understand, however, that this option is less effective than pulling your body through the water.)

For de-massing the lower body ...

To eliminate excess fat from your lower body–legs, stomach, waist, buttocks–develop a routine involving "legs-only" water exercises.

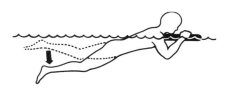

SWIMMERS: Rest your shoulders and arms on the board and propel yourself through the water by kicking your legs, using the flutter kick and/or frog kick. (These strokes are also fully described and illustrated later in this section.)

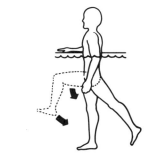

NON-SWIMMERS: Resting your shoulders and arms on the board while you perform "legs-only" exercises will keep your head above water. So will wearing a water jogging device as mentioned earlier.

Another option for nonswimmers is to stand in water reaching a few inches above the waist and perform "standing kicks"–standing frog kicks and/or knee raises–as detailed later in this section. Because these variations allow greater range of motion, they are at least as effective for de-massing as their counterparts involving a board.

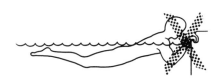

I don't recommend holding onto the edge of the pool or other stationary object while kicking; this position extracts effort from the upper body, thus reducing the effort extracted from the lower body.

Tip

For those at the intermediate to advanced level: Try capping off a legs-only routine with a few minutes of non-weighted sit backs, described on page 98, to enhance the session's effects.

For maintaining the target area ...

Once you achieve your de-massing and/or cardiorespiratory-strengthening goals, the most efficient way to maintain your new status is to use the same water exercises, but for shorter times and less often each week, to a minimum of two days a week. Alternatively, you can use appropriate floor exercises as discussed in Section 7. Floor exercises are also acceptable substitutes (albeit less effective ones) for those days when you can't work out in water. In any case, be sure to check your status frequently, as reflected by the mirror, not your scale.

For the Arms, Shoulders, Chest, back (Emphasis on chest):

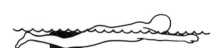

BREAST STROKE
(Arms Only)

Starting Position:

Lying prone in water holding board lightly between knees. Arms extended forward, backs of hands together. Face down in water.

Exercise Sequence:

1. Pull body through water via breast stroke arm motion:

    a) Lift head to breathe while pulling arms sideways through water until they are approximately at a 90-degree angle to body.

Getting It Together: Water Routines

b) Lowering face into water, draw elbows to sides of body, then return arms to starting position.

2. Repeat step 1 in smooth continuous motion until target muscles thoroughly fatigued. Do not extend water exercise session beyond 1-1/2 hours.

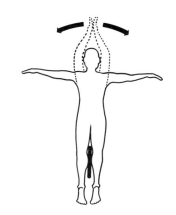

Common Pitfalls:

1. Allowing board to slip from between knees to between lower legs, reducing buoyancy provided by board and extracting unnecessary effort from leg muscles, reducing effectiveness of exercise on upper body.

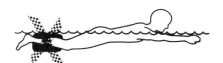

2. Gripping board too tightly with knees, extracting unnecessary effort from leg muscles and reducing effectiveness of exercise on upper body.

Tips:

1. NON-SWIMMERS can choose from three variations of this exercise:

    a) Hold head above water throughout exercise.
    b) Perform arm motion while standing or sitting in water deep enough to cover arms.
    c) Perform arm motion in deep water while wearing a water jogging device.

2. If you wish, you can combine other "arms-only" strokes with the breast stroke in a given session. Maintain each stroke for at least 12 minutes.

*For the Arms, Shoulders, Chest, Back
(Emphasis on arms and shoulders):*

AUSTRALIAN CRAWL
(Arms Only)

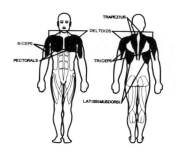

Starting Position:

Lying prone in water holding board lightly between knees. Lower part of face submerged, bridge of nose at water level. Arms extended forward, hands facing down.

Exercise Sequence:

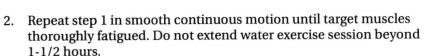

1. Pull body through water via Australian crawl arm motion:

   a) Draw one arm down and back through water until nearly pointed downward, gradually bending elbow.
   b) Lift elbow above water, then return arm to starting position.
   c) Simultaneously with b), rotate head to side (toward moving arm) until mouth above water for breathing, then return head to starting position.
   d) Perform steps a) and b) with other arm, initiating sequence as you complete b) with first arm.

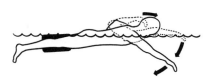

2. Repeat step 1 in smooth continuous motion until target muscles thoroughly fatigued. Do not extend water exercise session beyond 1-1/2 hours.

Common Pitfalls:

1. Allowing board to slip from between knees to between lower legs, reducing buoyancy provided by board and extracting unnecessary effort from leg muscles, reducing effectiveness of exercise on upper body.

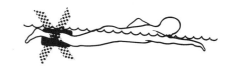

2. Gripping board too tightly with knees, extracting unnecessary effort from leg muscles and reducing effectiveness of exercise on upper body.

Tips:

1. NON-SWIMMERS can choose from three variations of this exercise:

    a) Hold head above water throughout exercise.
    b) Perform arm motion while standing or sitting in water deep enough to cover arms.
    c) Perform arm motion in deep water while wearing a water jogging device.

2. If you wish, you can combine other "arms-only" strokes with the Australian crawl in a given session. Maintain each stroke for at least 12 minutes.

For the Arms, Shoulders, Chest, Back (Emphasis on arms and shoulders):

BACKSTROKE
(Arms Only)

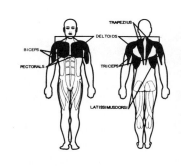

Starting Position:

Lying on back in water holding board lightly between knees. Arms at sides of body, hands facing down.

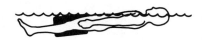

Exercise Sequence:

1. Pull body through water via backstroke arm motion:

    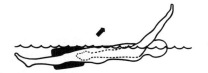

    a) Lift one arm up and back until it reaches water at about 10- or 2 o'clock position relative to body.
    b) Lower hand into water "pinkie" finger first until hand submerged 6-8 inches.
    c) Keeping thumb pointed up and hand submerged at same level, draw hand toward thigh.
    d) Repeat steps a) - c) with other arm.

2. Repeat step 1 in smooth continuous motion until target muscles thoroughly fatigued. Do not extend water exercise session beyond 1-1/2 hours.

Common Pitfalls:

1. Allowing board to slip from between knees to between lower legs, reducing buoyancy provided by board and extracting unnecessary effort from leg muscles, reducing effectiveness of exercise on upper body.

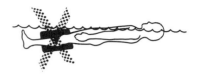

2. Gripping board too tightly with knees, extracting unnecessary effort from leg muscles and reducing effectiveness of exercise on upper body.

Tips:

1. NON-SWIMMERS should note that the face is not submerged during the backstroke. Alternatively, you can choose between two variations of this exercise:

    a) Perform arm motion while standing or sitting in water deep enough to cover arms.
    b) Perform arm motion in deep water while wearing a water jogging device.

2. If you wish, you can combine other "arms-only" strokes with the backstroke in a given session. Maintain each stroke for at least 12 minutes.

For the Thighs, Stomach, Buttocks:

FLUTTER KICKS
(Legs Only)

(This exercise helps prevent hamstring and thigh pulls related to activities requiring sprinting movement such as basketball fast breaks or track and field events.)

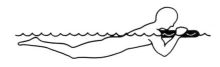

Starting Position:

Lying prone in water, shoulders supported by board. Arms bent and relaxed, hands resting on sides of board. Feet turned inward ("pigeon-toed"), toes pointed.

Exercise Sequence:

1. Exerting light pressure with hands to keep board about level, propel board through water via "flutter kick":

   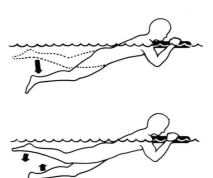

   a) Keeping leg straight, move one foot straight downward, then knee, then thigh. As hip is drawn into downward motion, it rotates, forcing other foot upward.
   b) Begin downward motion sequence with other foot simultaneously drawing first leg upward.
   c) Repeat steps a) and b) so that legs move up and down in opposition to each other, heels just reaching water surface.

2. Repeat step 1 in smooth continuous motion until target muscles thoroughly fatigued. Do not extend water exercise session beyond 1-1/2 hours.

Common Pitfalls:

1. Arms straight and extended with elbows locked, allowing upper body to participate and reducing effort extracted from thigh, stomach, and buttock muscles.

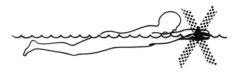

2. Feet facing downward or outward, or toes not pointed, reducing thrust created.

3. Beginning the kicking motion from hip or thigh muscles, reducing effort extracted from target muscles.

4. Kicking with lower legs only, reducing effort extracted from target muscles.

Tips:

1. NON-SWIMMERS: See "Standing Knee Lifts" later in this section, or perform this exercise in deep water while wearing a water jogging device.

2. When you first start this exercise, you may feel that only your legs are working. After about 5 minutes, you'll begin to feel the involvement of your stomach and buttock muscles.

3. If you wish, you can combine other "legs-only" strokes with flutter kicks in a given session. Maintain each stroke for at least 12 minutes.

For the Thighs, Stomach, Buttocks:

FROG KICKS
(Legs Only)

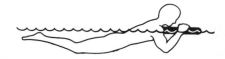

(This exercise helps prevent groin pulls related to activities requiring lateral movement such as tennis or racquetball.)

Starting Position:

Lying prone in water, shoulders supported by board. Arms bent and relaxed, hands resting on sides of board.

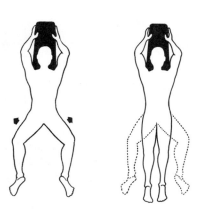

Exercise Sequence:

1. Exerting light pressure with hands to keep board about level, propel board through water via "frog kick":

    a) Bending knees forward and outward (pointed somewhat out from sides of body); draw feet toward body.
    b) Extend legs outward in easy motion, then pull legs together with more vigorous motion.

2. Repeat step 1 in smooth continuous motion until target muscles thoroughly fatigued. Do not extend water exercise session beyond 1-1/2 hours.

Common Pitfalls:

1. Arms straight and extended with elbows locked, allowing upper body to participate and reducing effort extracted from thigh, stomach, and buttock muscles.

2. Less-than-vigorous motion in pulling legs together, reducing effort extracted from target muscles.

3. Drawing legs together with knees, reducing effort extracted from target muscles and potentially stressing knee joints.

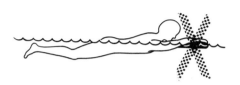

Tips:

1. NON-SWIMMERS: See "Standing Frog Kicks" later in this section. Perform this exercise in deep water while wearing a water jogging device.

2. When you first start this exercise, you may feel that only your legs are working. After about 5 minutes, you'll begin to feel the involvement of your stomach and buttock muscles.

3. If you wish, you can combine other "legs-only" strokes with frog kicks in a given session. Maintain each stroke for at least 12 minutes.

For the Thighs, Stomach, Buttocks:

STANDING KNEE LIFTS
(Legs Only)

(This Exercise helps prevent hamstring and thigh pulls related to activities requiring sprinting movement such as basketball fast breaks or field and track events. Due to the greater range of motion it allows, this exercise is even more effective in training for such events than flutter kicks with a board, and it's at least as effective for de-massing.)

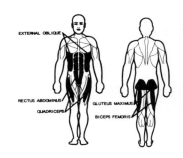

Starting Position:

Standing in water reaching a few inches above waist, hands on side of pool or other stationary object.

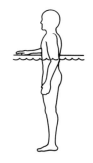

Exercise Sequence:

1. Perform "standing knee lifts":

   a) Lift one knee toward chest.
   b) In one continuous motion, return leg to starting position, then extend it as far backward as possible. Return leg to starting position.
   c) Repeat steps a) and b) with other leg.

2. Repeat step 1 until target muscles thoroughly fatigued. Do not extend water exercise session beyond 1-1/2 hours.

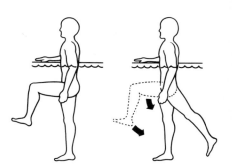

Common Pitfall:

Less-than-vigorous motion when moving leg down and back from raised position, reducing effort extracted from thigh, stomach, and buttock muscles.

Tips:

1. When you first start this exercise, you may feel that only your legs are working. After about 5 minutes, you'll begin to feel the involvement of your stomach and buttock muscles.

2. If you wish, you can combine other "legs-only" strokes with standing knee lifts in a given session. Maintain each stroke for at least 12 minutes.

For the Thighs, Stomach, Buttocks:

STANDING FROG KICKS
(Legs Only)

(This exercise helps prevent groin pulls related to activities requiring lateral movement such as tennis or racquetball. Due to the greater range of motion it allows, this exercise is even more effective in training for such events than frog kicks with a board, and it's at least as effective for de-massing.)

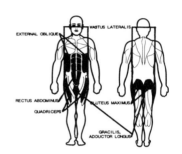

Starting Position:

Standing in water reaching a few inches above waist, hands on side of pool or other stationary object.

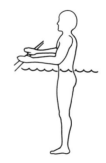

Exercise Sequence:

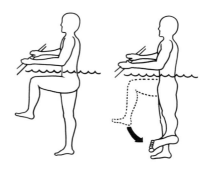

1. Perform "standing frog kicks":

   a) Bending one knee forward and outward (pointed somewhat out from sides of body), draw foot toward body.
   b) Extend leg outward in easy motion.
   c) Pull leg back to starting position with more vigorous motion.
   d) Repeat steps a) - c) with other leg.

2. Repeat step 1 until target muscles thoroughly fatigued. Do not extend water exercise session beyond 1-1/2 hours.

Common Pitfalls:

1. Less-than-vigorous motion when pulling leg back to starting position, reducing effort extracted from thigh, stomach, and buttock muscles.

2. Pulling leg back to starting position with knee, reducing effort extracted from target muscles and potentially stressing knee joint.

Tips:

1. When you first start this exercise, you may feel that only your legs are working. After about 5 minutes, you'll begin to feel the involvement of your stomach and buttock muscles.

2. If you wish, you can combine other "legs-only" strokes with standing frog kicks in a given session. Maintain each stroke for at least 12 minutes.

---

* The Wet Vest is from Bioenergetics, Inc., 5074 Shelby Dr., Birmingham, AL 35243, 205-991-8842. Flugels are produced by Barbara Huttner, Flugel Fitness, 4300 E. Mansfield Ave., Cherry Hills Village, Denver, CO 80237, 303-759-2882.

Chapter 6: Weight Room Routines; Anaerobic Exercises for Increasing, Strengthening Selected Muscles

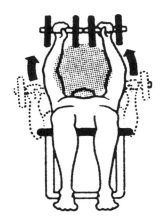

When your goal is to build and strengthen selected areas of your body, the idea is to work the muscles of that area until they are "pumped"–i.e., stressed to the point that blood rushes in and the adrenal gland secrets adrenaline/epinephrine hormone directly into the blood stream, that stimulates the heart, increases muscular strength and endurance. To maintain that "pump", work the muscles with short bursts of intense effort. (A "pumped" muscle becomes larger, tighter, and firmer to the touch.)

Such exercise is termed "anaerobic" because it enhances the muscles' ability to produce energy for movement without oxygen.

To produce changes in the muscles, you add resistance while you exercise, in the form of weights ranging from dumbbell and barbell weights to large, elaborate weight machines. Weight routines are usually performed in a specially-equipped weight room, most often at a gym or health spa; a number of "home" weight machines are available also.

For building strength and increasing muscle size, working with weights can't be beat. Exercising with weights entails its own special hazard, however. When people start working with weights and see those muscles developing, they're sometimes so delighted with the results that they begin to neglect the other components of their exercise program. Some people become so addicted to "pumping iron" that they do nothing else and end up in the very unhealthy situation of having big muscular bodies with cardio-respiratory systems that can no longer support their bodies and muscles that are no longer flexible.

> **Moral:**
> Don't neglect your aerobic exercise or your stretching while you work with weights. As your body becomes bigger and more muscular, it's crucial that your cardio-respiratory system grow stronger with it and that your muscles retain their flexibility.

How to Work With Weights

For building the target area ...

In a weight room session intended to build the target area, start with an amount of weight you can use in performing the exercise 10 times, comfortably but with some effort required toward the end of the sequence. Perform the exercise again with 5, 10, or 20 pounds more weight but with less repetitions, perhaps 8. Perform a total of five sets, increasing the weight and reducing the number of repetitions each time.

For example, the sequence might be:

Weight	Reps	
10 lbs.	10	
20 lbs.	8	(Sample only)
30 lbs.	6	
40 lbs.	4	
50 lbs.	1	

The two exceptions to this general rule of performing the exercises 10 reps with the starting weight, applies to the "Press Downs" exercise (page 112), and "Calf Raises" (page 119). Start these exercise with 15 repetitions using the starting weight.

A good rep pause count for all routines is the time it takes to say to yourself the number 1001.

After "maxing out" (performing the exercise once with the maximum weight), switch to your "rep out" weight and perform a rep out set by performing the exercise at least 5 but not more than 10 times. The rep out set brings additional blood supplies to the muscles.

When you're working one of the smaller muscle groups, your rep out weight can be 5, 10, or 20 pounds lighter than your starting weight. When a larger muscle group is being worked, your rep out weight can be 5, 10, or 20 pounds heavier than your starting weight. Experience will indicate the proper weight for you. In general, if you can't perform the exercise at least 5 times after maxing out, the weight's too heavy, and if you can perform it easily 10 times, it's too light.

After your rep out set, take a short break and move to the next exercise.

Some body builders use a technique called "flies" to enhance definition ("cuts") on muscle groups that are already increased and strengthened. This technique calls for lighter weights, a more limited range of motion, and a faster pace.

When using barbells, place your hands on the bar with the bar across the middle of your palms, not resting on the heel of your hand. Your hands should be approximately shoulder-width apart to ensure that your chest and shoulder muscles participate. If your hands are any closer, only your arm muscles will get any benefit from the exercise.

WARNING:

There is a real danger of straining, even pulling, muscles if you work out with too-heavy weights. When you start a weight lifting program, consult an instructor and be certain to start with, and increment by, appropriate weights. Further, bear in mind that what's "appropriate" for you can vary from day to day according to fluctuations in your health, how much sleep you got the night before, and so on. Recommended weight

increases are listed in the individual exercise descriptions in this section. Adjust these recommendations according to your particular status each day.

There's no particular recommended minimum amount of time for anaerobic exercise. From the following pages, you select the individual exercises that work the areas you wish to build. However long it takes to perform those exercises is the amount of time you need to spend.

On the other hand, there is very definitely a maximum time limit: you should complete an entire weight room session within an hour and a half, allowing for short breaks. Stop sooner in either of the following situations:

- You experience *any* pain or discomfort in a joint. Either you've overdone the exercise or you're doing it improperly. Consult an instructor before resuming that exercise.

- The target muscle loses its "pump" or becomes overfatigued.

If you're tempted to extend the session beyond an hour and a half, remember the dangers in doing so: overstressing the muscles, wearing down your body's immunities, and "burning out" on your program.

For toning the target area ...

You should use light to medium weight amounts at a higher rep count (15 to 20) for 5 sets and the fifth set's weight amount should drop to the rep out weight.

Whenever possible select joint supported weight room machines and routines.

For maintaining the target area ...

Once you've achieved your goal for a given area, you can maintain it with the same routine you used to reach that goal, but less often each week, down to a minimum of two days per week.

Section 7 describes floor exercises you can use for maintenance or as "at-home" substitutes when you're unable to get to the weight room.

For the Neck, Shoulders:

SHOULDER SHRUGS

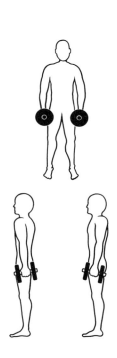

Starting Position:

Standing, starting weight in each hand, palms facing inward (toward body). Arms fully extended downward, held close to body.

Exercise Sequence:

1. Lift shoulders as high as possible and toward front, then lower shoulders to starting position.

2. Lift shoulders as high as possible and toward back. Hold for rep pause count 1001, then lower shoulders to starting position.

3. Repeat steps 1 and 2 to total this set's "rep count" (e.g., 10, 8, 6, 4, 1).

4. Increase weight by 10, 15, or 20 pounds. Repeat steps 1-3.

5. Repeat step 4 to total 5 sets.

6. After "maxing out," switch to "rep out" weight and perform exercise at least 5 but not more than 10 times.

7. Take a short break, then move to next exercise. Do not extend weight room session beyond 1-1/2 hours.

Common Pitfall:

Bending arms, increasing arm involvement and reducing effort extracted from shoulder muscles.

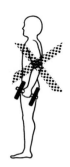

For the Shoulders:

MILITARY PRESSES

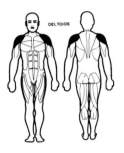

Starting Position:

Standing or sitting, starting weight in each hand, palms facing forward. Arms bent, elbows raised and pointed out from sides of body, weights touching shoulders.

Exercise Sequence:

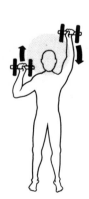

1. Slowly lift one weight upward until weight over head, hold for rep pause count 1001. (Envision a barrel resting on your chest; move arm accordingly.)

2. Lower weight to starting position while simultaneously lifting other weight as in step 1.

3. Repeat steps 1 and 2 to total this set's "rep count" (e.g., 10, 8, 6, 4, 1).

4. Increase weight by 10, 15, or 20 pounds. Repeat steps 1-3.

5. Repeat step 4 to total 5 sets.

6. After "maxing out," switch to "rep out" weight and perform exercise at least 5 but not more than 10 times.

7. Take a short break, then move to next exercise. Do not extend weight room session beyond 1-1/2 hours.

Common Pitfalls:

1. Snapping elbows, potentially stressing elbow joints.

2. Pointing elbows forward, increasing arm involvement and reducing effort extracted from shoulder muscles.

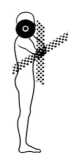

For the Chest, Triceps:

FLAT BENCH PULLOVER

(This is an exercise for stretching and warming up, primarily lower, middle chest and secondarily of Triceps, stretching and warming up these muscles will help enhance bench press, incline press, decline press, pull down and press down routines. The exercise calls for a spotter, someone strong enough to catch the weight if necessary. The spotter can also "boost" the weight slightly on the "max out" set.)

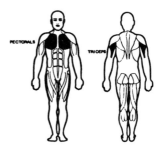

Starting Position:

Lying on back, starting weight in both hands, palms facing up. Arms straight up over the eyes.

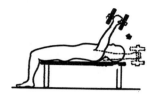

Exercise Sequence:

1. Keeping arms straight slowly lower the weight downward until arms are extended behind the head, parallel to the flat bench, hold for rep pause count 1001, then back to starting position.

2. Repeat step 1 to total this set's "rep count" (e.g., 10, 8, 6, 4, 1).

3. Increase weight by 10, 15 or 20 pounds. Repeat steps 1 and 2.

4. Repeat step 3 to total 5 sets.

5. "Maxing out"

6. Take a short break, then move to next exercise. Do not extend weight room session beyond 1 1/2 hours.

Common Pitfalls:

Positioning body perpendicular to the flat bench creating excessive pressure on neck and shoulders

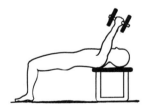

For the Middle Chest, Upper Arms:

FLAT BENCH PRESSES

(This is an exercise for building strength, primarily of the middle chest and secondarily of the upper and lower chest. Strengthening these muscles will help prevent dropping of the chest that sometimes comes with age. The exercise calls for a spotter, someone strong enough to catch the weight if necessary. The spotter can also "boost" the weight slightly on the "max out" set.)

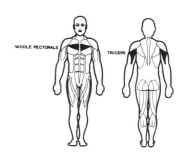

Starting Position:

Lying on back, starting weight in each hand, palms facing forward. Arms bent with elbows pointed out from sides of body. Weights touching shoulders.

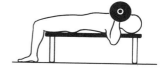

Exercise Sequence:

1. Keeping elbows pointed out to side, lift weights slowly upward until arms fully extended above eyes, hold for rep pause count 1001, then back to starting position. (Envision a large barrel resting on your chest; move arms accordingly.)

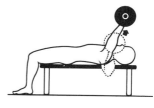

2. Repeat step 1 to total this set's "rep count" (e.g., 10, 8, 6, 4, 1).

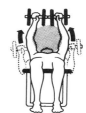

3. Increase weight by 10, 15, or 20 pounds. Repeat steps 1 and 2.

4. Repeat step 3 to total 5 sets.

5. After "maxing out," switch to "rep out" weight and perform exercise at least 5 but not more than 10 times.

6. Take a short break, then move to next exercise. Do not extend weight room session beyond 1-1/2 hours.

Common Pitfall:

Pointing elbows forward, increasing shoulder involvement and reducing effort extracted from middle chest and upper arm muscles.

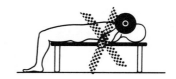

For the Upper Chest

INCLINE BENCH PRESSES

(This is an exercise for building strength, primarily of the upper chest and secondarily of the middle and lower chest. Strengthening these muscles will help prevent drooping of the chest that sometimes comes with age. The exercise calls for a spotter, someone strong enough to catch the weight if necessary. The spotter can also "boost" the weight slightly on the "max out" set.)

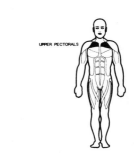

Starting Position:

Lying on back, starting weight in each hand, palms facing forward. Arms bent with elbows pointed out from sides of body. Weights touching shoulders.

Exercise Sequence:

1. Keeping elbows pointed out to side, lift weights slowly upward until arms fully extended above eyes. Hold for rep pause count 1001, then back to starting

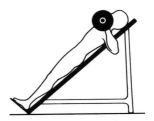

position. (Envision a large barrel resting on your chest; move arms accordingly.)

2. Repeat step 1 to total this set's "rep count" (e.g., 10, 8, 6, 4, 1).

3. Increase weight by 10, 15, or 20 pounds. Repeat steps 1 and 2.

4. Repeat step 3 to total 5 sets.

5. After "maxing out," switch to "rep out" weight and perform exercise at least 5 but not more than 10 times.

6. Take a short break, then move to next exercise. Do not extend weight room session beyond 1-1/2 hours.

Common Pitfall:

Pointing elbows forward, increasing shoulder involvement and reducing effort extracted from upper chest muscles.

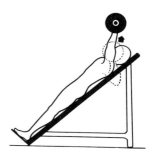

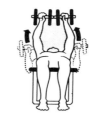

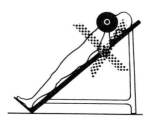

For the Lower Chest

DECLINE BENCH PRESSES

(This is an exercise for enhancing the size, shape, and contour of the lower chest–and thus its cosmetic appearance–and, secondarily, of the upper and middle chest. The exercise calls for a spotter, someone strong enough to catch the weight if necessary. The spotter can also "boost" the weight slightly on the "max out" set.)

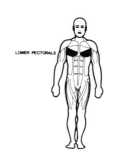

Getting It Together: Weight Room Routines

Starting Position:

Lying on back, starting weight in each hand, palms facing forward. Arms bent, elbows pointed out from sides of body. Weights touching shoulders.

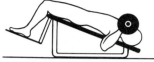

Exercise Sequence:

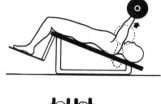

1. Keeping elbows pointed out to side, lift weights slowly upward until arms fully extended above eyes, hold for rep pause count 1001, then back to starting position. (Envision a large barrel resting on your chest; move arms accordingly.)

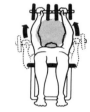

2. Repeat step 1 to total this set's "rep count" (e.g., 10, 8, 6, 4, 1).

3. Increase weight by 10, 15, or 20 pounds. Repeat steps 1 and 2.

4. Repeat step 3 to total 5 sets.

5. After "maxing out," switch to "rep out" weight and perform exercise at least 5 but not more than 10 times.

6. Take a short break, then move to next exercise. Do not extend weight room session beyond 1-1/2 hours.

Common Pitfall:

Pointing elbows forward, increasing shoulder involvement and reducing effort extracted from lower chest muscles.

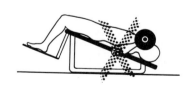

For the Back:

BEHIND-THE-NECK PULL DOWNS

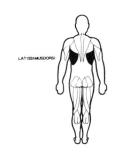

Starting Position:

Apparatus set with starting weight. Hands placed as wide as possible on apparatus bar, palms facing forward. Feet secured against apparatus base.

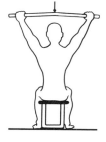

Exercise Sequence:

1. Pull bar down behind neck until it touches neck/shoulder area. Hold for rep pause count 1001, then return bar to starting position.

2. Repeat step 1 to total this set's "rep count" (e.g., 10, 8, 6, 4, 1).

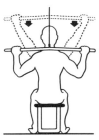

3. Increase weight by 10, 15, or 20 pounds. Repeat steps 1 and 2.

4. Repeat step 3 to total 5 sets.

5. After "maxing out," switch to "rep out" weight and perform exercise at least 5 but not more than 10 times.

6. Take a short break, then move to next exercise. Do not extend weight room session beyond 1-1/2 hours.

Common Pitfall:

Placing hands too close together on apparatus bar, increasing arm involvement and reducing effort extracted from back muscles.

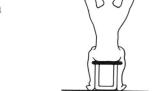

Getting It Together: Weight Room Routines

For the Upper Arms, Back Region:

PRESS DOWNS

(The triceps play a larger role in determining total arm strength than do the biceps.)

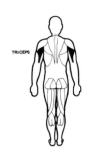

Starting Position:

Apparatus set with starting weight. Hands grasping apparatus bar on either side of supporting wire, bar across palms. Hands close together, palms facing down. Elbows bent, pressed against body.

Exercise Sequence:

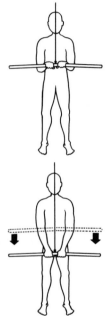

1. Press bar down until elbows lock, rotating knuckles downward just as elbows lock.

2. Hold bar down for rep pause count 1001, then return bar to starting position.

3. Repeat steps 1 and 2 to 11 to 10 total this set's "rep count" (e.g., 15, 10, 8, 4, 1). (Remember, 15 "reps," not 10, are recommended for the first set of this exercise.)

4. Increase weight by 5 or 10 pounds. Repeat steps 1-3.

5. Repeat step 4 to total 5 sets.

6. After "maxing out," switch to "rep out" weight and perform exercise at least 5 but not more than 10 times.

7. Take a short break, then move to next exercise. Do not extend weight room session beyond 1-1/2 hours.

Common Pitfalls:

1. Holding elbows away from body, increasing shoulder involvement and reducing effort extracted from triceps.

2. Placing hands too far apart on bar, increasing shoulder involvement and reducing effort extracted from triceps.

3. Rolling shoulders, increasing shoulder involvement and reducing effort extracted from triceps.

4. Resting bar on heels of hands, preventing rotation of knuckles and reducing effort extracted from triceps.

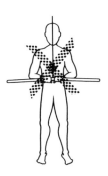

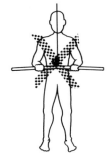

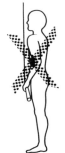

For the Upper Arms, Front Region:

SUPPORTED CURLS

Starting Position:

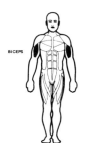

Sitting, starting weight in one hand, palm facing upward. Arm fully extended downward and supported at the middle of the triceps either by other arm (as illustrated) or by "preacher bench."

Exercise Sequence:

1. Bending arm at elbow, lift weight toward body until it touches shoulder. Hold for rep pause count 1001, then lower arm to starting position.

2. Repeat step 1 to total this set's "rep count" (e.g., 10, 8, 6, 4, 1).

3. Increase weight by 5 pounds. Repeat steps 1 and 2.

4. Repeat step 3 to total 5 sets.

5. After "maxing out," switch to "rep out" weight and perform exercise at least 5 but not more than 10 times.

6. Take a short break, then switch weight to other hand and repeat steps 1-5.

7. Take a short break, then move to next exercise. Do not extend weight room session beyond 1-1/2 hours.

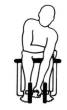

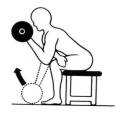

Common Pitfall:

"Working" arm not properly supported, allowing movement other than flexing, which decreases effort extracted from biceps. The most common form of this pitfall results from placing the hand of the supporting arm on the wrong thigh, as shown.

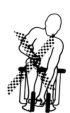

For the Stomach:

WEIGHTED SIT BACKS

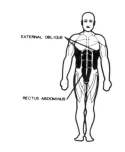

Starting Position:

Sitting on flat bench. Hands holding starting weight (dumbbell) behind head.

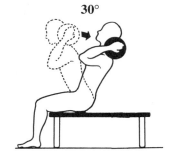

Exercise Sequence:

1. Lean back until stomach muscles begin to work to support upper body. Hold as long as possible.

2. Twist upper body to the right, back to center, to the left, back to center. Repeat until fatigued, hold for rep pause count 1001, then return to starting position.

3. Repeat steps 1 and 2 to total this set's "rep count" (e.g., 10, 8, 6, 4, 1).

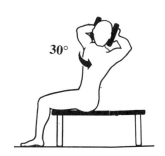

4. Increase weight by 10, 15, or 20 pounds. Repeat steps 1-3.

5. Repeat step 4 to total 5 sets.

6. After "maxing out," switch to "rep out" weight and perform exercise at least 5 but not more than 10 times.

7. Take a short break, then move to next exercise. Do not extend weight room session beyond 1-1/2 hours.

Common Pitfall:

Failing to keep stomach muscles pulled in, causing them to develop in "pushed out" position.

Tip:

1. If necessary, omit barbell plate and clasp hands behind head when starting to do this exercise.

For the Thighs and :buttocks

WEIGHTED THREE-QUARTER SQUATS

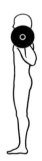

Starting Position:

Standing, starting barbell weight supported on shoulders. Feet about hip-width apart, toes pointed straight forward (to work inner quadriceps and inner buttocks).

Exercise Sequence:

1. Keeping back straight, bend forward slightly and lower body to about 3/4 of full squat. Hold for rep count 1001, then raise body to starting position.

2. Repeat step 1 to total this set's "rep count" (e.g., 10, 8, 6, 4, 1).

3. Increase weight by 10, 15, or 20 pounds. Repeat steps 1 and 2.

4. Repeat step 3 to total 5 sets.

5. After "maxing out," switch to "rep out" weight and perform exercise at least 5 but not more than 10 times.

6. Take a short break, then move feet to shoulder-width and point toes slightly outward (to work outer quadriceps and outer buttocks). Repeat steps 1-5.

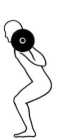

7. Take a short break, then move to next exercise. Do not extend weight room session beyond 1-1/2 hours.

Common Pitfall:

Lowering body to full squat position, placing all of the weighted pressure on the knee joint region of the thigh muscle. This type of misapplied weighted pressure causes loosening of the knee joint from the supporting thigh muscle group, resulting in a condition commonly called a "trick knee." (The 3/4 squat places the weighted pressure squarely on the main portion of the mid-thigh muscle group.)

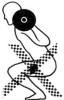

The full squat exercise is a required event in power lifting events. The 3/4 squat is a more productive exercise for enhancing leg strength and stamina for events involving running or kicking action such as football or soccer.

Tip:

I don't recommend attempting this exercise with your toes pointed inward (i.e., "pigeon-toed") or outward, as these positions are very awkward. Studies have shown that placing the feet straight forward will prevent unnecessary stress on ankle, knee and hip joints and supporting muscle groups.

For the Hamstrings, Buttocks:

LEG CURLS

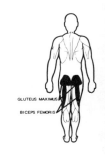

Starting Position:

Apparatus set with starting weight. Lying on stomach, feet beneath rollers attached to weights.

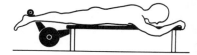

Exercise Sequence:

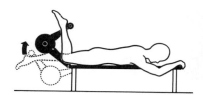

1. Bend knees and slowly lift lower legs until nearly perpendicular to body. Hold for rep pause count 1001, then back to starting position.

2. Return legs to starting position. Rest for 2 seconds.

3. Repeat steps 1 and 2 to total this set's "rep count" (e.g., 10, 8, 6, 4, 1).

4. Increase weight by 5 or 10 pounds. Repeat steps 1-3.

5. Repeat step 4 to total 5 sets.

6. After "maxing out," switch to "rep out" weight and perform exercise at least 5 but not more than 10 times.

7. Take a short break, then move to next exercise. Do not extend weight room session beyond 1-1/2 hours.

Common Pitfall:

Lifting legs beyond perpendicular, placing all of the weighted pressure on the knee joint region of the thigh muscle. This type of misapplied weighted pressure causes loosening of the knee joint from the supporting thigh muscle group, resulting in a condition commonly called a "trick knee."

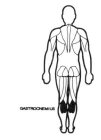

For the Calves:

WEIGHTED CALF RAISES

Starting Position:

Apparatus set with starting weight. Standing on apparatus base, toes pointed straight forward, rear portion of feet extended over edge.

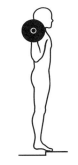

Exercise Sequence:

1. Keeping back and knees straight, lift body as high as possible, then lower body as far as possible.

2. Repeat step 1, hold for rep pause count 1001, then return to starting position.

3. Repeat steps 1 and 2 to total this set's "rep count" (e.g., 15, 15, 15, 15, 10).

4. Increase weight by 10, 15, or 20 pounds. Repeat sets 1-3.

5. Repeat step 4 to total 5 sets.

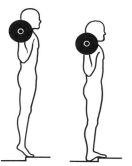

6. After "maxing out," switch to "rep out" weight and perform exercise at least 5 but not more than 10 times.

7. Take a short break, then move feet so toes point outward. Repeat steps 1-6.

8. Take a short break, then move to next exercise. Do not extend weight room session beyond 1-1/2 hours.

Common Pitfall:

Bending knees, increasing thigh muscle involvement and reducing effort extracted from calf muscles.

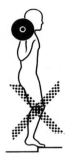

Chapter 7: Floor Exercises;
Aerobic or Anaerobic Exercises For Maintenance, At-Home Substitutes

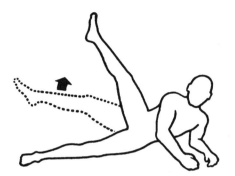 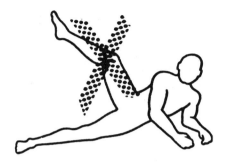

The exercises described in this section do not require weights or other equipment and thus can be performed at home. Floor exercises are best performed on a gym mat or similar surface, but a carpeted floor is fine. Your comfort is all that matters.

In general, try to perform each exercise until the target muscles are thoroughly fatigued–not just "pretty tired" but not overly stressed either. Do not extend the session beyond an hour and a half, for all the reasons stated earlier.

How To Perform Floor Exercises

For Maintenance ...

When you use floor exercises for maintenance, devise a routine made up of exercises from the following pages that work the areas you wish to maintain. Stop each exercise as soon as the target muscles become "pumped" or overly fatigued. At least two days per week are required for maintenance.

As Substitutes For Water or Weight Room Routines ...

When you're confined indoors for the day–for whatever reason - you can substitute appropriate exercises from the following pages for your normal water and/or weight room routine. Bear in mind, however, that floor exercise substitutes are at best pale imitations of their weight room or water counterparts. Use them as substitutes *only* when you really don't have any other choice.

When you substitute floor exercises for a water routine, perform them aerobically, that is, with your heart rate elevated to the proper level and for a minimum of 12 minutes.

For Aerobic Value ...

If you need to add aerobic exercise to an otherwise all-anaerobic workout schedule, you can use selected floor exercises to provide that aerobic value. Simply perform those exercises at a sufficient pace to raise your heart rate to the appropriate rate and maintain that rate for at least 12 minutes.

Be sure, however, to choose exercises that don't conflict with the rest of your program–i.e., that don't work the areas you're trying to build up.

For the Shoulders:

ARM TWIRLS

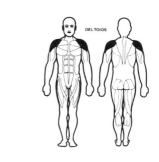

Starting Position:

Standing, feet about hip-width apart. Arms and hands at shoulder level, fully extended straight out from sides of body.

Exercise Sequence:

1. Move hands and arms in 4 to 6 inch circles until arms begin to fatigue.

2. Reverse direction of circles. Repeat step 1.

3. Repeat steps 1 and 2 as long as possible.

4. Take a short break, then move to next exercise. Do not extend floor exercise session beyond 1-1/2 hours.

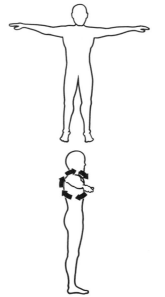

Common Pitfall:

Allowing arms to drop below shoulder level, reducing effort extracted from shoulder muscles.

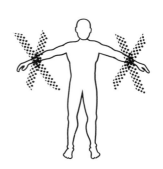

Getting It Together: Floor Exercises

Tips:

1. To enhance this exercise, either wear wrist weights or hold weights of some sort in your hands.

2. For slight variations in the muscles worked by this exercise, use any of the following modifications. (Maintain each variation for at least a full minute.)

    a). Hold hands with fingers pointed outward, then down, then up, then fists clenched.
    b). Vary circle size from small to medium to large.

For the Neck, Shoulders:

SHOULDER SHRUGS

Starting Position:

Standing, arms fully extended downward, held close to body.

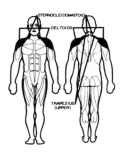

Exercise Sequence:

1. Lift shoulders as high as possible and toward front, then lower shoulders to starting position.

2. Lift shoulders as high as possible and toward back, then lower shoulders to starting position.

3. Repeat steps 1 and 2 until fatigued.

4. Take a short break, then move to next exercise. Do not extend floor exercise session beyond 1-1/2 hours.

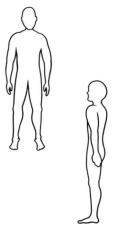
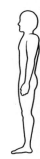

Getting It Together: Floor Exercises

Common Pitfall:

Bending arms, increasing arm involvement and reducing effort extracted from shoulder muscles.

Tip:

To enhance this exercise, either wear wrist weights or hold weights of some sort in your hands.

For the Arms, Shoulders:

CHIN UPS

Starting Position:

Grasping chinning bar, hands shoulder-width apart, palms facing forward. (Isn't every home equipped with a chinning bar?)

Exercise Sequence,
Emphasis on Shoulders:

1. Lift body with head behind bar until chin level with bar, then lower body not quite to fully lowered (i.e., arms slightly bent).

2. Lift body with head in front of bar until bar touches neck/shoulder area, the lower body not quite to fully lowered (i.e., arms slightly bent).

3. Repeat steps 1 and 2 until fatigued.

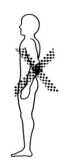
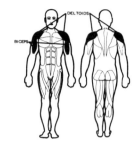
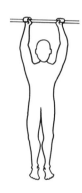
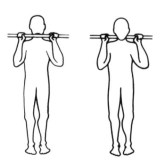

4; Take a short break, then move to next exercise. Do not extend floor exercise session beyond 1-1/2 hours.

Exercise Sequence, Emphasis on Arms:

Steps outlined on preceding page, *except*:

1. Grasp bar with hands *less than* shoulder-width apart.

2. Lower body *fully* (i.e., arms straight).

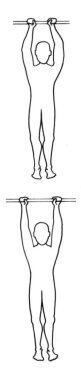

For the Upper Arms, Chest:

PUSH UPS - 1

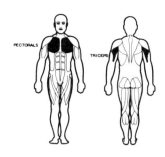

Starting Position:

On hands and knees, hands shoulder-width apart, fingers pointed forward. Hands moved forward, upper body shifted forward until upper body forms level plane between shoulders and area just above knee caps, weight centered on arms and area just above knee caps. Feet raised and (optionally) crossed.

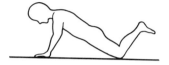

Exercise Sequence:

1. Keeping back level, lower body nearly to floor, then back up to starting position.

2. Repeat step 1 until fatigued.

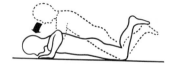

3. Take a short break, then move to next exercise. Do not extend floor exercise session beyond 1-1/2 hours.

Common Pitfalls:

1. Lowering just upper body, reducing effort extracted from arm and chest muscles.

2. Raising buttocks above level plane between shoulders and knees, reducing effort extracted from arm and chest muscles.

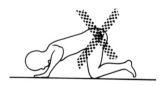

Getting It Together: Floor Exercises

Tip:

For slight variations in the muscles worked by this exercise, use any of the following variations. (Maintain each variation for at least a full minute.)

1. Point fingers forward, then outward to side, then inward (toward each other).

2. Place hands at shoulder-width, then closer together.

3. To focus the effort more on the arm muscles than on the chest muscles, place hands further than shoulder-width apart.

For the Upper Arms, Chest:

PUSH UPS - 2

WARNING!

If the upper body lacks sufficient strength. Use "Push-Ups - 1" to increase upper body strength before attempting this exercise routine again.

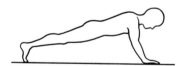

Starting Position:

Hands shoulder-width apart, fingers pointed forward. Legs extended, body lifted until it forms level plane between shoulders and feet. Weight supported by hands and balls of feet.

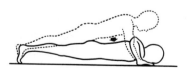

Exercise Sequence:

1. Keeping back level, lower body nearly to floor, then back up to starting position.

2. Repeat step 1 until fatigued.

3. Take a short break, then move to next exercise. Do not extend floor exercise session beyond 1-1/2 hours.

Common Pitfalls:

1. Lowering just upper body, reducing effort extracted from arm and chest muscles.

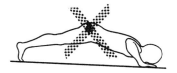

2. Raising buttocks above level plane between shoulders and knees, reducing effort extracted from arm and chest muscles.

Tip:

For slight variations in the muscles worked by this exercise, use any of the following variations. (Maintain each variation for at least a full minute.)

1. Point fingers forward, then outward to side, then inward (toward each other).

2. Place hands at shoulder width, then closer together.

3. To focus the effort more on the arm muscles than on the chest muscles, place hands further than shoulder-width apart.

Getting It Together: Floor Exercises

For the Stomach:

SIT BACKS

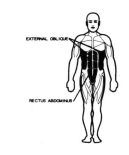

Starting Position:

Sitting on floor or flat bench. Hands clasped behind head.

Exercise Sequence:

1. Lean back until stomach muscles begin to work to support upper body. Hold position as long as possible.

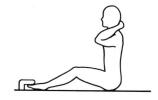

2. Twist upper body to the right, back to center, to the left, back to center.

3. Repeat step 2 until fatigued, then return to starting position.

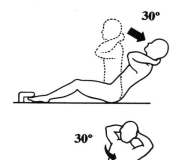

4. Take a short break, then move to next exercise. Do not extend floor exercise session beyond 1-1/2 hours.

Common Pitfall:

Failing to keep stomach muscles pulled in, causing them to develop in "pushed out" position.

Tip:

1. When you reach the intermediate to advanced level, you'll find that a few minutes of this exercise following a legs-only water routine enhances the session's de-massing effects.

For the Buttocks:

HIP RAISES

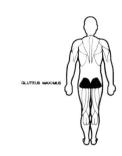

Starting Position:

Lying on back, arms relaxed along sides of body. Knees bent. Feet hip-width apart 8-10 inches from buttocks. Hips raised to form even plane from knees to head.

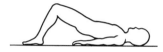

Exercise Sequence:

1. Clenching buttock muscles tightly, raise hips as high as possible.

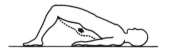

2. Relax buttock muscles and lower hips to starting position.

3. Repeat steps 1 and 2 until fatigued.

4. Clenching buttock muscles tightly, raise hips as high as possible. Hold as long as possible.

5. Lower hips to starting position, then to floor.

6. Take a short break, then move to next exercise. Do not extend floor exercise session beyond 1-1/2 hours.

Getting It Together: Floor Exercises

Common Pitfalls:

1. Failing to clench buttock muscles tightly, reducing effort extracted.

2. Lowering hips below starting position, an unnecessary and nonproductive motion.

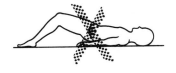

For the Thighs, Buttocks:

THREE-QUARTER SQUATS

Starting Position:

Standing, feet about hip-width apart, toes pointed straight forward.

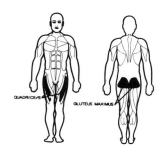

Exercise Sequence:

1. Keeping back straight, bend forward slightly and lower body to about 3/4 of full squat. Hold position for 2 seconds, then raise body to starting position.

2. Repeat step 1 until fatigued.

3. Take a short break, then move feet to shoulder-width and point toes slightly outward (to work outer thighs and outer buttocks). Repeat steps 1 and 2.

4. Take a short break, then move to next exercise. Do not extend floor exercise session beyond 1-1/2 hours.

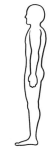

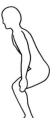

Getting It Together: Floor Exercises

Tip:

I don't recommend attempting this exercise with your toes pointed inward (i.e., "pigeon-toed") or outward, as these positions are very awkward. Studies have shown that placing the feet straight forward will prevent unnecessary stress on ankle, knee and hip joints and supporting muscle groups.

Common Pitfall:

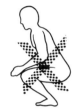

Lowering body to full squat position, placing all of the pressure on the knee joint region of the thigh muscle. This type of misapplied pressure causes loosening of the knee joint from the supporting thigh muscle group, resulting in a condition commonly called a "trick knee." (The 3/4 squat places the pressure squarely on the main portion of the mid-thigh muscle group.)

The full squat exercise is a required event in power lifting events. The 3/4 squat is a more productive exercise for increasing leg strength and stamina for events requiring running or kicking action such as football or soccer.

For the Thighs:

LEG LIFTS

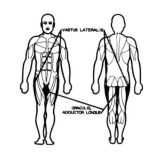

Starting Position:

Lying on side, one leg on top of other.

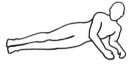

Exercise Sequence:

1. Keeping legs straight, lift upper leg toward ceiling and then as far as possible toward head in a smooth constant motion without moving leg toward front or rear, then lower leg to starting position.

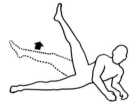

2. Repeat step 1 until fatigued.

3. Change sides, repeat steps 1 and 2.

4. Take a short break, then move to next exercise. Do not extend floor exercise session beyond 1-1/2 hours.

Common Pitfalls:

1. "Throwing" leg rather than lifting it, reducing effort extracted from thigh muscles.

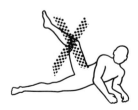

2. Bending knee, increasing buttocks involvement and reducing effort extracted from thigh muscles.

Tips:

1. To increase the difficulty (and thus the effectiveness) of this exercise, raise lower leg 4-5 inches off floor. In this position, the upper leg works harder and the lower leg works as well.

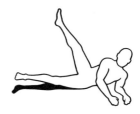

2. For slight variations in the muscles worked by this exercise, use any of the following modifications. (Maintain each variation for at least a full minute).

    a). Flex foot, then point toes.
    b). Lift leg straight upward, then toward front, then toward rear.

For the Calves:

CALF RAISES

Starting Position:

Standing on low raised surface, toes pointed straight forward, rear portion of feet extended over edge.

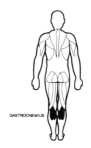

Exercise Sequence:

1. Keeping back and knees straight, lift body as high as possible, then lower body as far as possible, then return to starting position.

2. Repeat step 1 until fatigued.

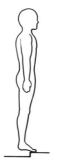

Getting It Together: Floor Exercises

3. Take a short break, then adjust feet so toes point outward. Repeat steps 1-3.

4. Take a short break, then move to next exercise. Do not extend floor exercise session beyond 1-1/2 hours.

Common Pitfall:

Bending knees, increasing thigh muscle involvement and reducing effort extracted from calf muscles.

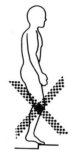

Appendix

Recommended Reading

Anatomical Kinesiology. Jerry N. Barham and William L. Thomas. The Macmillian Co., Toronto, Ontario, Canada. 1969.

Essential Human Anatomy. James E. Crouch. Lea & Ferbiger, Philadelphia, PA. 1981.

Exercise Physiology. William P. McArdle, Frank I. Katch, and Victor L. Katch. Lea & Ferbiger, Philadelphia, PA. 1981.

Fit or Fat? Covert Bailey. Houghton Mifflin Co., Boston, MA. 1977.

Stretching. Bob Anderson. Shelter Publications, Inc., Bolinas, CA. 1980.

About the Author

John Ireland is a practitioner of the concepts he outlines in this book.

Heavily involved in sports throughout high school and college (football, rugby, baseball), he was exposed early to traditional sports training methods and has continued with a fitness program ever since. Studies in physiology, nutrition, kinesiology, and related subjects lead to a bachelor's degree in physical education from San Diego State University in 1976.

After sixteen years of doing all the "right" things and not getting all the results he wanted, he developed alternative and supplementary techniques. They've worked for him 6...4 and for everyone else who has learned them. He realized that this approach could be helpful to virtually anyone, and the result was this book.

John's Exercise History
After years of experimenting with various weekly workout schedules, John finally settled on a program that started to close the gap on his short and long term goals.

This schedule was targeted at separating the routines into upper and lower body sessions. Monday, Wednesday, and Friday were spent in the weight room working on building the upper body. Tuesday and Thursday were intended to reduce the lower body and were spent running distances, doing sit ups, and attending aerobics classes.

It was a "good" schedule, by most yardsticks, and the lower body work was showing the results he'd been seeking. However, it became apparent that he wasn't going to totally eliminate the "love handles," bulging tummy and backside, and oversized legs with this program. Further, he felt that his Tuesday and Thursday exertions taxed his energies for the Wednesday and Friday workouts.

So, he looked around for other avenues that would more efficiently isolate and concentrate his efforts to eliminate areas of unwanted fat, and found the solution in a swimming pool. Continuing to lift weights two days a week to maintain the upper body, he began using a "legs-only" water routine with a board three days a week.

Some time later, he worked with a group of "non-swimmers" who had some difficulty mastering the board routines, and developed alternative techniques done standing or sitting in water. He found these variations to be just as effective for de-massing and even more effective as training for athletic events, so he switched his personal "legs-only" water workout from a board routine to a standing routine.

Once he had achieved his de-massing goals, he added weight room routines to his schedule to build and strengthen his lower body.

Currently, Monday and Wednesday involve about 20 minutes in the pool plus some 10 minutes in the weight room for maintaining the lower body. Tuesday and Thursday are weight room sessions of about 45 minutes for maintaining the upper body. Friday, Saturday, and Sunday are for enjoying the results.

As a high-tech manufacturer's sales representative for the past 10 years, John is no stranger to business-related stress flare-ups. When such flare-ups occured, he'd find that many of his muscles were tensed. He'd also notice that he was taking shallow breaths through his mouth rather than breathing normally (and more productively) through his nose. These reactions, common to many people under stress, cause improper blood oxygen transfer and thus improper cell nourishment throughout the body.

Of course, the most constructive way to deal with stress is to correct whatever is causing it. All too often, however, the stress-inducer is beyond our control. Powerless to do anything about the cause of the stress, we're left with all its negative effects.

John has found that exercising is a positive way to deal with those negative effects. By forcing concentration on proper breathing techniques and on the movements associated with the routine, a physical workout alleviates the physical manifestations of the stress, clears the mind of the anxiety and stressful thoughts that tagged along into the session, and creates a sense of having control. In John's case, it's a sense of having control over making his sales. For others, it might be a sense of having control over resolving a family crisis, solving a financial difficulty, or surmounting the next hurdle, whatever it may be.

This fresh outlook and sense of having control stems from knowing that the anxiety and stress have been dealt with in a positive way; we all need continual positive reinforcement regarding our actions.

A physical workout leaves us better equipped both mentally and physically to attain our goals. Other popular stress reducers like alcohol, tobacco, or drugs, on the other hand, can only leave a dulled sense of what those goals were in the first place.

A Page From John's Photo Album ...

↙ ME!

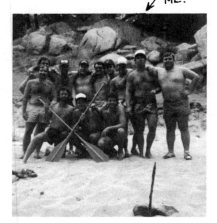

The infamous "belly" shot. Taken the day before I started the three-days-a-week "legs-only" pool routine.

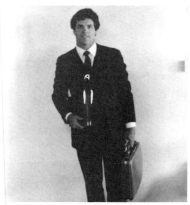

Beginning to see a little better fit to the suit ...

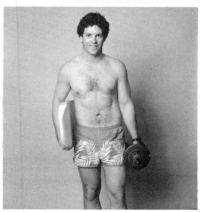

... and now a little definition in the stomach ...

... and now a fair amount of definition! (These pictures taken two months after I started the standing "legs-only" routines in the pool.) Photos by John Balik.

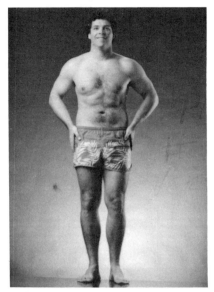
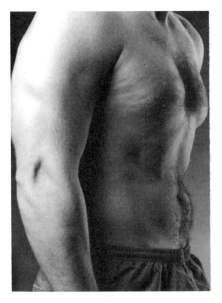
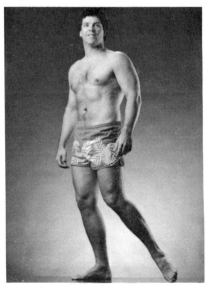
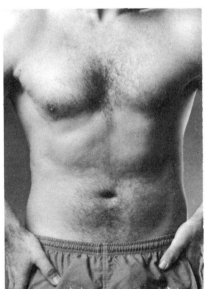

Appendix

These pictures show the results two months after I combined the standing "Leg–Only" routine with weight room stomach and leg routines. Photos by John Post.

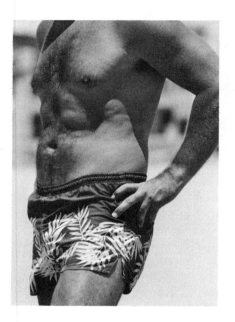
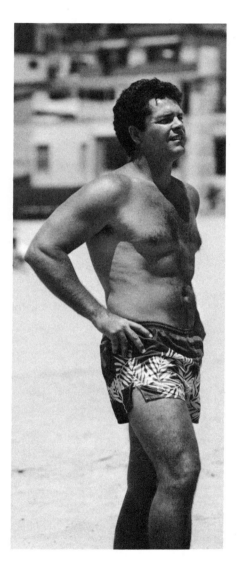

Index

A

acids 56
adrenaline 99
aerobic
　43, 64, 69, 76, 77, 81, 121
aerobic dancing 40, 41
aerobic exercise 40, 43
aging 40, 47
alcohol 55
amino 56
anaerobic 43, 64, 99, 102, 121
ankle 81
ankles 40
apple 55, 57
arm 51
ARM TWIRLS 123
Arms 86, 88, 90, 107, 112, 113
arms 41, 50, 125, 127, 128
arteriosclerosis 55
AUSTRALIAN CRAWL 88
avocados 54

B

back 81, 86, 88, 90, 111
BACKSTROKE 90
beans 56
BEHIND-THE-NECK PULL
　DOWNS 111
belly 42
biceps
　AUSTRALIAN CRAWL 88
　BACKSTROKE 90
　BREAST STROKE 86
　CHIN UPS 125
　SUPPORTED CURLS 113

biceps femoris
　FLUTTER KICKS 92
　LEG CURLS 118
　STANDING KNEE LIFTS 96
biotin 56
blood 55, 67, 99
blood vessels 55
bloodstream 54, 55
bonding 55
brain 56
bread 46
BREAST STROKE 86
breath 50
breathing 40, 44, 75
burn-outs 76
burning fat 41
buttock 41
buttocks
　42, 71, 92, 94, 96, 97, 116, 118,
　131, 132

C

caffeine 55
calcium 56
CALF RAISES 119, 135
caloric 45, 56
calorie 46
calories 59
calves 119, 135
capillaries 55
carbohydrate 56
carbohydrates 46, 59, 63
carbon dioxide 55
carboxyl 56
cardiorespiratory
　40, 64, 67, 72, 81, 83, 100

Appendix

carrot 57
caviar 55
celery 57
cells 57
cellulite 51, 81
cheeseburger 62
chemical 67
chest
   67, 86, 88, 90, 105, 107, 127, 128
CHIN UPS 125
cholesterol 56
choline 57
citrus 57
CO_2 55
Complex carbohydrates 54
conversion 56
cuts 101

D

dairy 56
dairy products 54
de-mass 42, 81
De-Massing 44, 64, 67
DECLINE BENCH PRESSES 109
dehydration 59
deltoid
  ARM TWIRLS 123
  AUSTRALIAN CRAWL 88
  BACKSTROKE 90
  BREAST STROKE 86
  CHIN UPS 125
  MILITARY PRESSES 104
  SHOULDER SHRUGS 103, 124
diet 46, 55
diets 59
dressings 58
drinking 59
drinks 55

E

eating 40, 55, 57, 63
eating habits 47, 51
egg yolks 55
electrolyte 59
endorphin 56
energy 44, 62
enzymes 40, 46
epinephine 99
exhale 75
external oblique
  FLUTTER KICKS 92
  FROG KICKS 94
  SIT BACKS 130
  STANDING FROG KICKS 97
  STANDING KNEE LIFTS 96
  WEIGHTED SIT BACKS 115

F

face 40, 45
fast 58
fat 40, 45, 55, 64, 81
  excess 42
  unwanted 43
fatigue 41, 56, 75, 82
fatigued 83, 87, 90, 102, 121
Fats 54
fats 56
Fatty foods 54
fish 54, 56
FLAT BENCH PRESSES 107
FLAT BENCH PULLOVER 105
flexibility 100
flies 101
Floor Exercises 121
Flugels 84
FLUTTER KICKS 92
folacin 56
Food and drug 57
foods
  fatty 54

Appendix

frog kick 43
FROG KICKS 94
fruits 54, 57

G

gastrocnemius
   CALF RAISES 135
   WEIGHTED CALF RAISES 119
glucose 56
gluteus maximus
   FLUTTER KICKS 92
   FROG KICKS 94
   HIP RAISES 131
   LEG CURLS 118
   STANDING FROG KICKS 97
   STANDING KNEE LIFTS 96
   THREE-QUARTER SQUATS 132
   WEIGHTED THREE-QUARTER
      SQUATS 116
gout 55
gracilis adductor longus 94
   LEG LIFTS 134
   STANDING FROG KICKS 97
grains 54, 57
gross aerobic exercise 40, 41

H

hamstring 96
Hamstrings 118
headedness 56
heart 41, 50, 99
heart rate
   40, 44, 59, 69, 71, 77, 122
heavy legs 42
HIP RAISES 131
hormone 99
hydrogen 55
hydrolysis 56
hypoglycemia 56

I

INCLINE BENCH PRESSES 108
infated belts 45
inhale 75
intramuscular 45
iodine 57
iron 57

J

jacuzzi 82
jogging 40, 41, 69
joint 102
joints 81
jugular vein 78
juice 59
jumping jacks 40

K

"kick in" 44
knee 81
knees 40

L

lactic acid 75
Large muscle 41
latissimusdorsi
   AUSTRALIAN CRAWL 88
   BACKSTROKE 90
   BEHIND-THE-NECK PULL
      DOWNS 111
   BREAST STROKE 86
LEG CURLS 118
LEG LIFTS 134
leg muscles 43
legs 50, 51
   heavy 42
legumes 56
levels
   cholesterol 55
   uric 55

lift weights 47
ligaments 40
   torn 40
liquids 59
liver 55
love handles 42, 51, 71
Lower Body 67
lower body 41, 64, 85

M

M., Patrick McGrady 54
magnesium 56
Maintenance 64, 68, 121
meats 54, 55
metabolic 57
metabolism 41
   carbohydrate 54
MILITARY PRESSES 104
Minerals 56
minerals 56
mirror 46, 50, 63
Miss Manner 58
morphine 56
Muscle 70
muscle 64, 75
   large 41
   small 41
muscles 81, 99, 101, 121
   ability 40
   different 43
   leg 43

N

neck 41, 103, 124
niacin 56
nuts 54

O

oils 54
oily vegetables 54
oranges 55

overweight 56
oxygen 44, 55, 75, 81

P

pasta 46, 54, 58
pectorals
   AUSTRALIAN CRAWL 88
   BACKSTROKE 90
   BREAST STROKE 86
   DECLINE BENCH PRESSES 109
   FLAT BENCH PRESSES 107
   FLAT BENCH PULLOVER 105
   INCLINE BENCH PRESSES 108
   PUSH UPS - 1 127
   PUSH UPS - 2 128
peppers 57
peptides 56
potassium 57, 59
potatoes 46
poultry 56
PRESS DOWNS 112
Pritikin, Nathan 54
protein 55
proteins 46
pumped 76, 99, 122
PUSH UPS - 1 127
PUSH UPS - 2 128

Q

quadriceps
   FLUTTER KICKS 92
   FROG KICKS 94
   STANDING FROG KICKS 97
   STANDING KNEE LIFTS 96
   THREE-QUARTER SQUATS 132
   WEIGHTED THREE-QUARTER
      SQUATS 116

R

rectus abdominius
   SIT BACKS 130

STANDING FROG KICKS 97
STANDING KNEE LIFTS 96
WEIGHTED SIT BACKS 115
rectus abdominus
   FLUTTER KICKS 92
   FROG KICKS 94
rice 54
running 40, 41, 43, 66, 69

S

salad 57
salt 55
sauce 58
saunas 45
scale 46, 55, 63
shin 81
SHOULDER SHRUGS 103, 124
Shoulders
    41, 86, 88, 90, 103, 104, 123, 124, 125
shrimp 55
SIT BACKS 115, 130
size 64, 100
skipping rope 40, 69
small muscle 41
spine 40
sports bottle 59
Spot Reducing 45
sprints 66
stamina 40, 41, 50, 51, 71
STANDING FROG KICKS 97
STANDING KNEE LIFTS 96
starches 59
sternocleidomastoid
   SHOULDER SHRUGS 103, 124
stomach
    51, 67, 71, 75, 92, 94, 96, 97, 115, 130
strength 71, 99
strengthen 81, 83
strengthening 64, 67

stress 44, 67
stress fractures 40
stressed 56, 81, 99, 121
Stretching 70
subcutaneous 46
sugar 55, 59
sundae 62
SUPPORTED CURLS 113
sweat suits 45
Swimming 40
swimming 41, 43
swimming pool 42
system
   cardioespiratory 44

T

tendinitis 40
thigh 41, 51
   inner and outer 43
Thighs
    71, 92, 94, 96, 97, 116, 132, 134
thirsty 59
THREE-QUARTER SQUATS
    116, 132
thyroid 57
tissues 55, 56
tomatoes 57
toxins 56
trapezius
   AUSTRALIAN CRAWL 88
   BACKSTROKE 90
   BREAST STROKE 86
   SHOULDER SHRUGS 103, 124
treadmill 50
Triceps 105
triceps
   AUSTRALIAN CRAWL 88
   BACKSTROKE 90
   BREAST STROKE 86
   FLAT BENCH PRESSES 107
   FLAT BENCH PULLOVER 105

   PRESS DOWNS 112
   PUSH UPS - 1 127
   PUSH UPS - 2 128
tubers 56

U

upper body 41, 64, 67, 84
uric levels 55

V

vastus lateralis
   FROG KICKS 94
   LEG LIFTS 134
   STANDING FROG KICKS 97
vegetable 56
vegetables 54
Vitamins 56

W

waist 51
Warm Up 76
water 55, 59, 81, 84
water routines 43
Weight 99
weight lifting 42, 43
weight routines 45
weights 47, 81
Wet Vest 84
Women 47

Y

YMCA 82
YWCA 82

Z

zero impact 81

ORDER FORM

Please send me the following:

_____   copies of <u>Getting It Together!</u> @ $14.95:

plus shipping and handling:

_____ $4.50 book rate surface mail worldwide

_____ $6.00 book rate air mail United States, Canada, Mexico

_____ $8.00 book rate air mail elsewhere

California residents please add 8.25% sales tax: _____

Total Enclosed: _____

Name: _____

Street: _____

City/State/Zip _____

Country _____

When ordering from outside the United States, please make payment in the form of a postal money order, a check drawn on a bank with an agent in the United States, or an international money order, payable in U.S. dollars.

Mail form with payment made out to John Ireland to:
    John Ireland
    401 Manhattan Beach Blvd.
    Manhattan Beach, CA 90266
    U.S.A.

Exercise Log Sheets

Following are monthly log sheets which you can use to outline your personal exercise program and to record your adherence to it.

First enter your name and the month on the top line, and number the days to correspond to the month in question. Then select *your* exercises from the "Activity" list at the left of the sheet. If you've chosen any weight room exercises, fill in the weight amounts and number of repetitions. (Each weight room exercise calls for five sets with increasing weights and decreasing repetitions, plus a rep out set.) Enter the numbers of the selected exercises in the appropriate slots.

On each day you follow through with your program and do the scheduled exercises, mark the "Ck" box with an "X" or a check mark (Maybe a gold star?)

_____'S WORKOUT SCHEDULE FOR _____
(name) (month)

ACTIVITY

WATER
1. BREAST STROKE
2. AUSTRALIAN CRAWL
3. BACKSTROKE
4. FLUTTER KICKS
5. FROG KICKS
6. STANDING KNEE LIFTS
7. STANDING FROG KICKS

FLOOR
8. ARM TWIRLS
9. SHOULDER SHRUGS
10. CHIN UPS
11. PUSH-UPS - 1
12. PUSH-UPS - 2
13. SIT BACKS
14. HIP RAISES
15. 3/4 SQUATS
16. LEG LIFTS
17. CALF RAISES

WEIGHT ROOM
18. MILITARY PRESSES
    WT:
    RP:
19. SHOULDER SHRUGS
    WT:
    RP:
20. SUPPORTED CURLS
    WT:
    RP:
21. PRESS DOWNS
    WT:
    RP:
22. PULLDOWNS
    WT:
    RP:
23. FLAT BENCH PULLOVER
    WT:
    RP:
24. INCLINE BENCH PRESSES
    WT:
    RP:
25. FLAT BENCH PRESSES
    WT:
    RP:
26. DECLINE BENCH PRESSES
    WT:
    RP:
27. SIT BACKS
    WT:
    RP:
28. 3/4 SQUATS
    WT:
    RP:
29. LEG CURLS
    WT:
    RP:
30. CALF RAISES
    WT:
    RP:

	SUNDAY Date / Ck.	MONDAY Date / Ck.	TUESDAY Date / Ck.	WEDNESDAY Date / Ck.	THURSDAY Date / Ck.	FRIDAY Date / Ck.	SATURDAY Date / Ck.

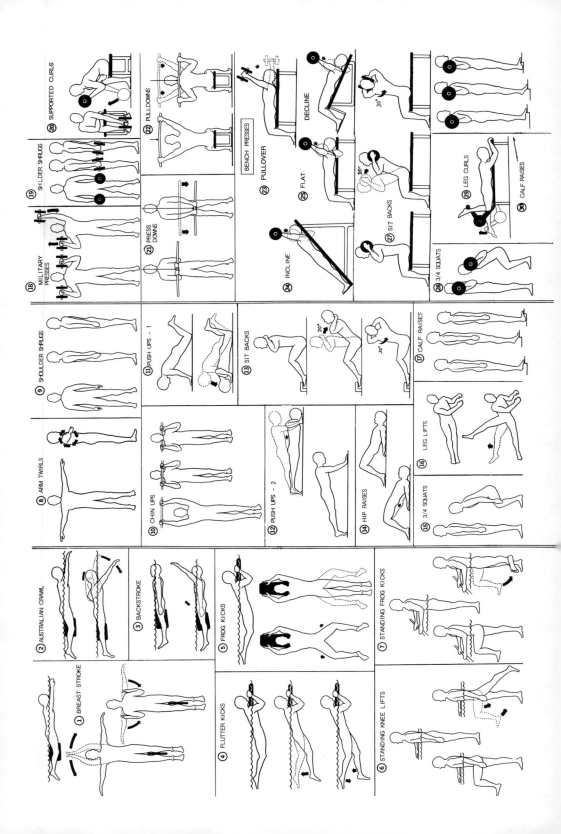

_____'S WORKOUT SCHEDULE FOR _____

(name) (month)

ACTIVITY	SUNDAY Date / Ck.	MONDAY Date / Ck.	TUESDAY Date / Ck.	WEDNESDAY Date / Ck.	THURSDAY Date / Ck.	FRIDAY Date / Ck.	SATURDAY Date / Ck.

WATER
1. BREAST STROKE
2. AUSTRALIAN CRAWL
3. BACKSTROKE
4. FLUTTER KICKS
5. FROG KICKS
6. STANDING KNEE LIFTS
7. STANDING FROG KICKS

FLOOR
8. ARM TWIRLS
9. SHOULDER SHRUGS
10. CHIN UPS
11. PUSH-UPS - 1
12. PUSH-UPS - 2
13. SIT BACKS
14. HIP RAISES
15. 3/4 SQUATS
16. LEG LIFTS
17. CALF RAISES

WEIGHT ROOM
18. MILITARY PRESSES
    WT:
    RP:
19. SHOULDER SHRUGS
    WT:
    RP:
20. SUPPORTED CURLS
    WT:
    RP:
21. PRESS DOWNS
    WT:
    RP:
22. PULLDOWNS
    WT:
    RP:
23. FLAT BENCH PULLOVER
    WT:
    RP:
24. INCLINE BENCH PRESSES
    WT:
    RP:
25. FLAT BENCH PRESSES
    WT:
    RP:
26. DECLINE BENCH PRESSES
    WT:
    RP:
27. SIT BACKS
    WT:
    RP:
28. 3/4 SQUATS
    WT:
    RP:
29. LEG CURLS
    WT:
    RP:
30. CALF RAISES
    WT:
    RP:

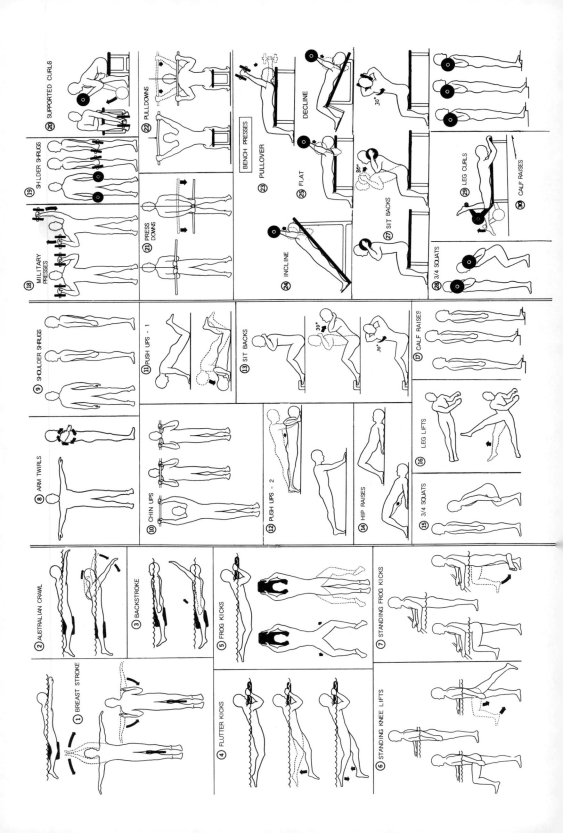

_____'S WORKOUT SCHEDULE FOR _____

(name)   (month)

ACTIVITY

WATER
1. BREAST STROKE
2. AUSTRALIAN CRAWL
3. BACKSTROKE
4. FLUTTER KICKS
5. FROG KICKS
6. STANDING KNEE LIFTS
7. STANDING FROG KICKS

FLOOR
8. ARM TWIRLS
9. SHOULDER SHRUGS
10. CHIN UPS
11. PUSH-UPS - 1
12. PUSH-UPS - 2
13. SIT BACKS
14. HIP RAISES
15. 3/4 SQUATS
16. LEG LIFTS
17. CALF RAISES

WEIGHT ROOM

18. MILITARY PRESSES
WT:
RP:

19. SHOULDER SHRUGS
WT:
RP:

20. SUPPORTED CURLS
WT:
RP:

21. PRESS DOWNS
WT:
RP:

22. PULLDOWNS
WT:
RP:

23. FLAT BENCH PULLOVER
WT:
RP:

24. INCLINE BENCH PRESSES
WT:
RP:

25. FLAT BENCH PRESSES
WT:
RP:

26. DECLINE BENCH PRESSES
WT:
RP:

27. SIT BACKS
WT:
RP:

28. 3/4 SQUATS
WT:
RP:

29. LEG CURLS
WT:
RP:

30. CALF RAISES
WT:
RP:

	SUNDAY Date / Ck.	MONDAY Date / Ck.	TUESDAY Date / Ck.	WEDNESDAY Date / Ck.	THURSDAY Date / Ck.	FRIDAY Date / Ck.	SATURDAY Date / Ck.

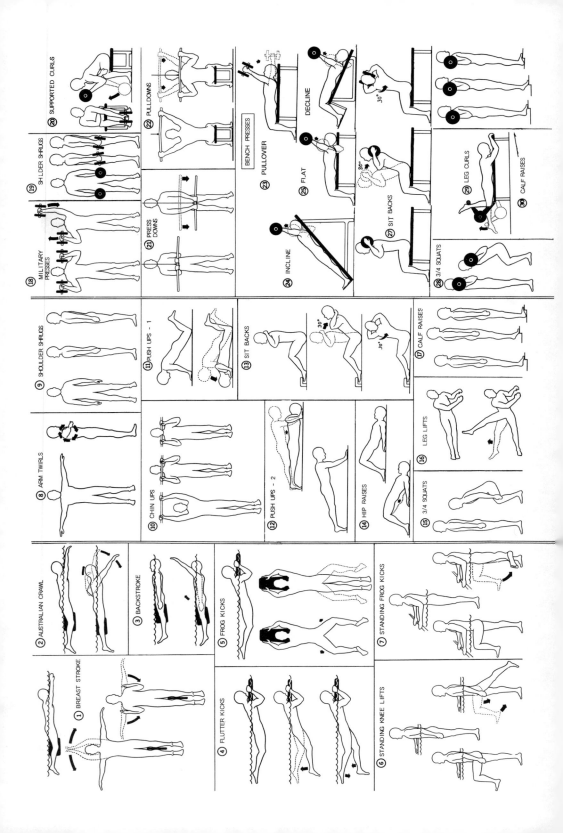

_____'S WORKOUT SCHEDULE FOR _____

(name) (month)

ACTIVITY

WATER
1. BREAST STROKE
2. AUSTRALIAN CRAWL
3. BACKSTROKE
4. FLUTTER KICKS
5. FROG KICKS
6. STANDING KNEE LIFTS
7. STANDING FROG KICKS

FLOOR
8. ARM TWIRLS
9. SHOULDER SHRUGS
10. CHIN UPS
11. PUSH-UPS - 1
12. PUSH-UPS - 2
13. SIT BACKS
14. HIP RAISES
15. 3/4 SQUATS
16. LEG LIFTS
17. CALF RAISES

WEIGHT ROOM

18. MILITARY PRESSES
WT:
RP:

19. SHOULDER SHRUGS
WT:
RP:

20. SUPPORTED CURLS
WT:
RP:

21. PRESS DOWNS
WT:
RP:

22. PULLDOWNS
WT:
RP:

23. FLAT BENCH PULLOVER
WT:
RP:

24. INCLINE BENCH PRESSES
WT:
RP:

25. FLAT BENCH PRESSES
WT:
RP:

26. DECLINE BENCH PRESSES
WT:
RP:

27. SIT BACKS
WT:
RP:

28. 3/4 SQUATS
WT:
RP:

29. LEG CURLS
WT:
RP:

30. CALF RAISES
WT:
RP:

	SUNDAY Date / Ck.	MONDAY Date / Ck.	TUESDAY Date / Ck.	WEDNESDAY Date / Ck.	THURSDAY Date / Ck.	FRIDAY Date / Ck.	SATURDAY Date / Ck.

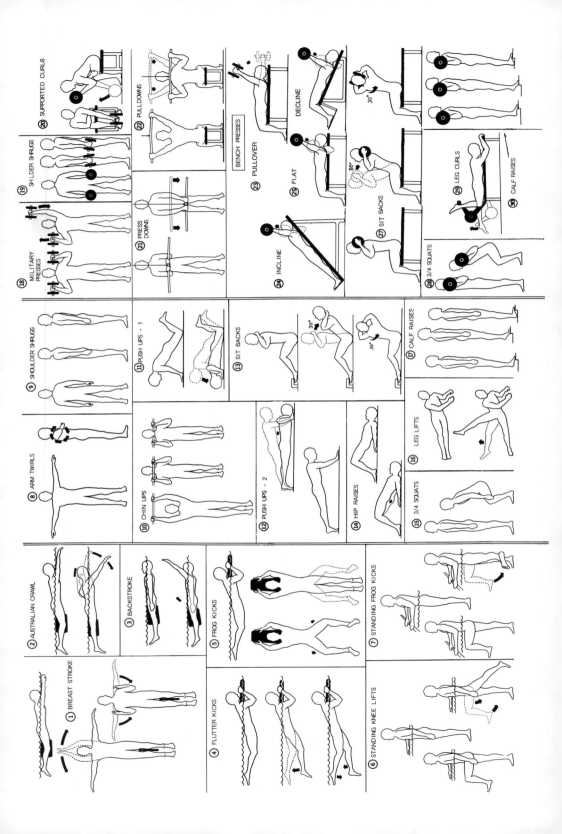

_____'S WORKOUT SCHEDULE FOR _____
(name) (month)

ACTIVITY		SUNDAY Date / Ck.	MONDAY Date / Ck.	TUESDAY Date / Ck.	WEDNESDAY Date / Ck.	THURSDAY Date / Ck.	FRIDAY Date / Ck.	SATURDAY Date / Ck.

WATER
1. BREAST STROKE
2. AUSTRALIAN CRAWL
3. BACKSTROKE
4. FLUTTER KICKS
5. FROG KICKS
6. STANDING KNEE LIFTS
7. STANDING FROG KICKS

FLOOR
8. ARM TWIRLS
9. SHOULDER SHRUGS
10. CHIN UPS
11. PUSH-UPS - 1
12. PUSH-UPS - 2
13. SIT BACKS
14. HIP RAISES
15. 3/4 SQUATS
16. LEG LIFTS
17. CALF RAISES

WEIGHT ROOM

18. MILITARY PRESSES
    WT:
    RP:

19. SHOULDER SHRUGS
    WT:
    RP:

20. SUPPORTED CURLS
    WT:
    RP:

21. PRESS DOWNS
    WT:
    RP:

22. PULLDOWNS
    WT:
    RP:

23. FLAT BENCH PULLOVER
    WT:
    RP:

24. INCLINE BENCH PRESSES
    WT:
    RP:

25. FLAT BENCH PRESSES
    WT:
    RP:

26. DECLINE BENCH PRESSES
    WT:
    RP:

27. SIT BACKS
    WT:
    RP:

28. 3/4 SQUATS
    WT:
    RP:

29. LEG CURLS
    WT:
    RP:

30. CALF RAISES
    WT:
    RP:

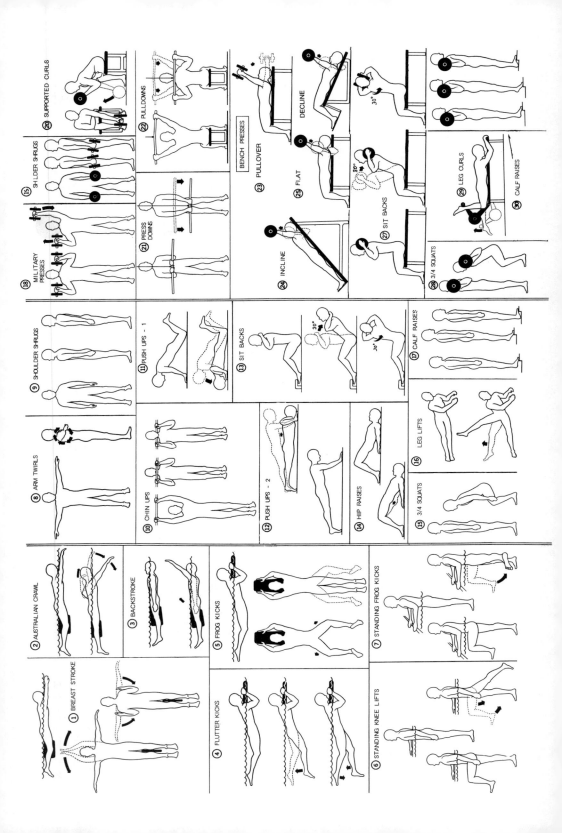

_____'S WORKOUT SCHEDULE FOR _____

(name)   (month)

ACTIVITY	SUNDAY Date/Ck.	MONDAY Date/Ck.	TUESDAY Date/Ck.	WEDNESDAY Date/Ck.	THURSDAY Date/Ck.	FRIDAY Date/Ck.	SATURDAY Date/Ck.

WATER
1. BREAST STROKE
2. AUSTRALIAN CRAWL
3. BACKSTROKE
4. FLUTTER KICKS
5. FROG KICKS
6. STANDING KNEE LIFTS
7. STANDING FROG KICKS

FLOOR
8. ARM TWIRLS
9. SHOULDER SHRUGS
10. CHIN UPS
11. PUSH-UPS - 1
12. PUSH-UPS - 2
13. SIT BACKS
14. HIP RAISES
15. 3/4 SQUATS
16. LEG LIFTS
17. CALF RAISES

WEIGHT ROOM
18. MILITARY PRESSES
   WT: ____
   RP: ____
19. SHOULDER SHRUGS
   WT: ____
   RP: ____
20. SUPPORTED CURLS
   WT: ____
   RP: ____
21. PRESS DOWNS
   WT: ____
   RP: ____
22. PULLDOWNS
   WT: ____
   RP: ____
23. FLAT BENCH PULLOVER
   WT: ____
   RP: ____
24. INCLINE BENCH PRESSES
   WT: ____
   RP: ____
25. FLAT BENCH PRESSES
   WT: ____
   RP: ____
26. DECLINE BENCH PRESSES
   WT: ____
   RP: ____
27. SIT BACKS
   WT: ____
   RP: ____
28. 3/4 SQUATS
   WT: ____
   RP: ____
29. LEG CURLS
   WT: ____
   RP: ____
30. CALF RAISES
   WT: ____
   RP: ____

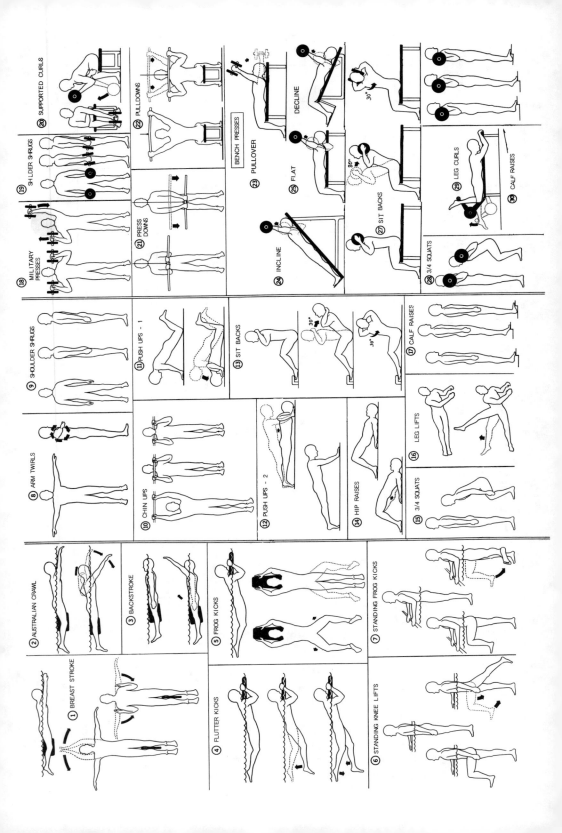

_____'S WORKOUT SCHEDULE FOR _____

(name)   (month)

ACTIVITY

WATER
1. BREAST STROKE
2. AUSTRALIAN CRAWL
3. BACKSTROKE
4. FLUTTER KICKS
5. FROG KICKS
6. STANDING KNEE LIFTS
7. STANDING FROG KICKS

FLOOR
8. ARM TWIRLS
9. SHOULDER SHRUGS
10. CHIN UPS
11. PUSH-UPS - 1
12. PUSH-UPS - 2
13. SIT BACKS
14. HIP RAISES
15. 3/4 SQUATS
16. LEG LIFTS
17. CALF RAISES

WEIGHT ROOM

18. MILITARY PRESSES
WT:
RP:

19. SHOULDER SHRUGS
WT:
RP:

20. SUPPORTED CURLS
WT:
RP:

21. PRESS DOWNS
WT:
RP:

22. PULLDOWNS
WT:
RP:

23. FLAT BENCH PULLOVER
WT:
RP:

24. INCLINE BENCH PRESSES
WT:
RP:

25. FLAT BENCH PRESSES
WT:
RP:

26. DECLINE BENCH PRESSES
WT:
RP:

27. SIT BACKS
WT:
RP:

28. 3/4 SQUATS
WT:
RP:

29. LEG CURLS
WT:
RP:

30. CALF RAISES
WT:
RP:

	SUNDAY Date / Ck.	MONDAY Date / Ck.	TUESDAY Date / Ck.	WEDNESDAY Date / Ck.	THURSDAY Date / Ck.	FRIDAY Date / Ck.	SATURDAY Date / Ck.

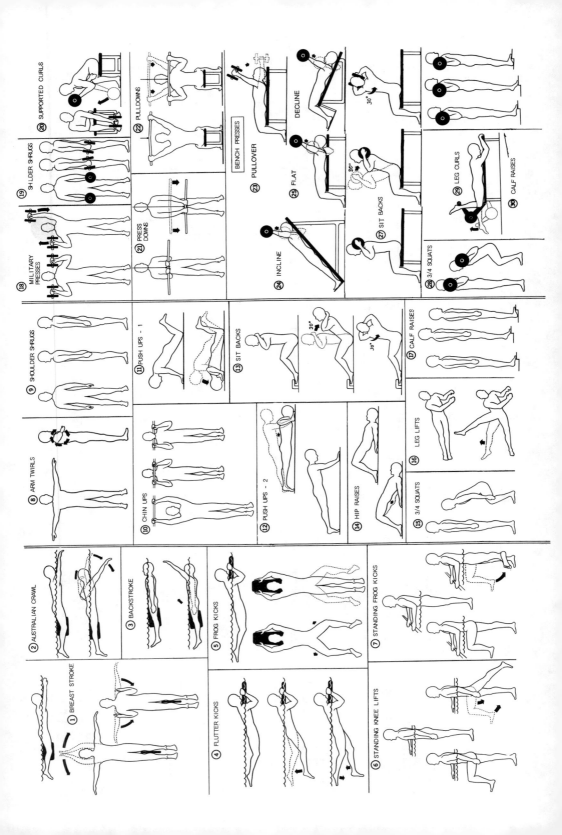

_____'S WORKOUT SCHEDULE FOR _____
(name)   (month)

ACTIVITY

WATER
1. BREAST STROKE
2. AUSTRALIAN CRAWL
3. BACKSTROKE
4. FLUTTER KICKS
5. FROG KICKS
6. STANDING KNEE LIFTS
7. STANDING FROG KICKS

FLOOR
8. ARM TWIRLS
9. SHOULDER SHRUGS
10. CHIN UPS
11. PUSH-UPS - 1
12. PUSH-UPS - 2
13. SIT BACKS
14. HIP RAISES
15. 3/4 SQUATS
16. LEG LIFTS
17. CALF RAISES

WEIGHT ROOM

18. MILITARY PRESSES
    WT:
    RP:
19. SHOULDER SHRUGS
    WT:
    RP:
20. SUPPORTED CURLS
    WT:
    RP:
21. PRESS DOWNS
    WT:
    RP:
22. PULLDOWNS
    WT:
    RP:
23. FLAT BENCH PULLOVER
    WT:
    RP:
24. INCLINE BENCH PRESSES
    WT:
    RP:
25. FLAT BENCH PRESSES
    WT:
    RP:
26. DECLINE BENCH PRESSES
    WT:
    RP:
27. SIT BACKS
    WT:
    RP:
28. 3/4 SQUATS
    WT:
    RP:
29. LEG CURLS
    WT:
    RP:
30. CALF RAISES
    WT:
    RP:

	SUNDAY Date / Ck.	MONDAY Date / Ck.	TUESDAY Date / Ck.	WEDNESDAY Date / Ck.	THURSDAY Date / Ck.	FRIDAY Date / Ck.	SATURDAY Date / Ck.

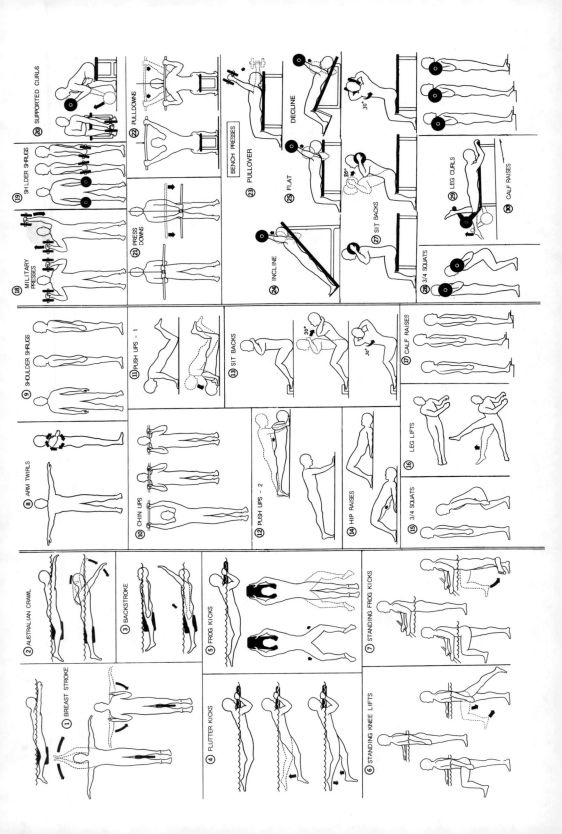

_____'s WORKOUT SCHEDULE FOR _____
(name)   (month)

ACTIVITY

WATER
1. BREAST STROKE
2. AUSTRALIAN CRAWL
3. BACKSTROKE
4. FLUTTER KICKS
5. FROG KICKS
6. STANDING KNEE LIFTS
7. STANDING FROG KICKS

FLOOR
8. ARM TWIRLS
9. SHOULDER SHRUGS
10. CHIN UPS
11. PUSH-UPS - 1
12. PUSH-UPS - 2
13. SIT BACKS
14. HIP RAISES
15. 3/4 SQUATS
16. LEG LIFTS
17. CALF RAISES

WEIGHT ROOM
18. MILITARY PRESSES — WT: ___ RP: ___
19. SHOULDER SHRUGS — WT: ___ RP: ___
20. SUPPORTED CURLS — WT: ___ RP: ___
21. PRESS DOWNS — WT: ___ RP: ___
22. PULLDOWNS — WT: ___ RP: ___
23. FLAT BENCH PULLOVER — WT: ___ RP: ___
24. INCLINE BENCH PRESSES — WT: ___ RP: ___
25. FLAT BENCH PRESSES — WT: ___ RP: ___
26. DECLINE BENCH PRESSES — WT: ___ RP: ___
27. SIT BACKS — WT: ___ RP: ___
28. 3/4 SQUATS — WT: ___ RP: ___
29. LEG CURLS — WT: ___ RP: ___
30. CALF RAISES — WT: ___ RP: ___

	SUNDAY Date / Ck.	MONDAY Date / Ck.	TUESDAY Date / Ck.	WEDNESDAY Date / Ck.	THURSDAY Date / Ck.	FRIDAY Date / Ck.	SATURDAY Date / Ck.

Get into it! Get into Together

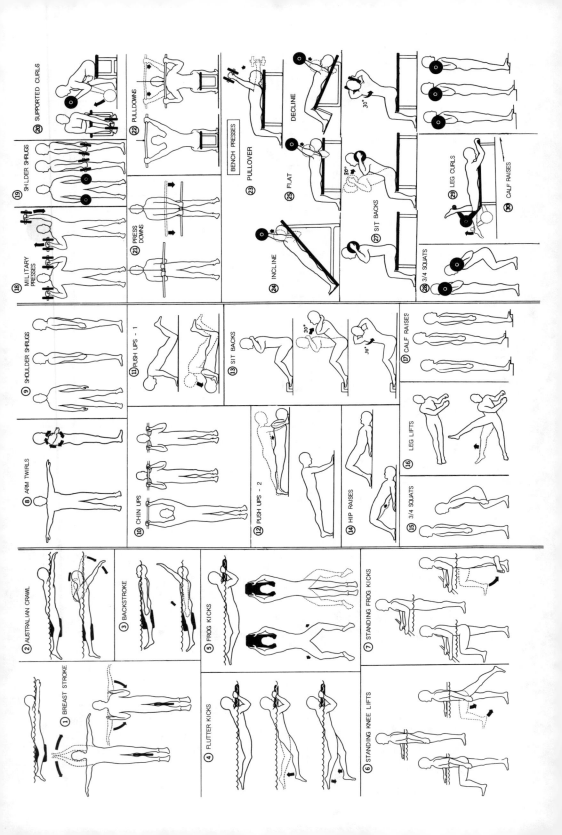

_____'s WORKOUT SCHEDULE FOR _____

(name)   (month)

	SUNDAY Date / Ck.	MONDAY Date / Ck.	TUESDAY Date / Ck.	WEDNESDAY Date / Ck.	THURSDAY Date / Ck.	FRIDAY Date / Ck.	SATURDAY Date / Ck.

ACTIVITY

WATER
1. BREAST STROKE
2. AUSTRALIAN CRAWL
3. BACKSTROKE
4. FLUTTER KICKS
5. FROG KICKS
6. STANDING KNEE LIFTS
7. STANDING FROG KICKS

FLOOR
8. ARM TWIRLS
9. SHOULDER SHRUGS
10. CHIN UPS
11. PUSH-UPS - 1
12. PUSH-UPS - 2
13. SIT BACKS
14. HIP RAISES
15. 3/4 SQUATS
16. LEG LIFTS
17. CALF RAISES

WEIGHT ROOM

18. MILITARY PRESSES
    WT:
    RP:
19. SHOULDER SHRUGS
    WT:
    RP:
20. SUPPORTED CURLS
    WT:
    RP:
21. PRESS DOWNS
    WT:
    RP:
22. PULLDOWNS
    WT:
    RP:
23. FLAT BENCH PULLOVER
    WT:
    RP:
24. INCLINE BENCH PRESSES
    WT:
    RP:
25. FLAT BENCH PRESSES
    WT:
    RP:
26. DECLINE BENCH PRESSES
    WT:
    RP:
27. SIT BACKS
    WT:
    RP:
28. 3/4 SQUATS
    WT:
    RP:
29. LEG CURLS
    WT:
    RP:
30. CALF RAISES
    WT:
    RP:

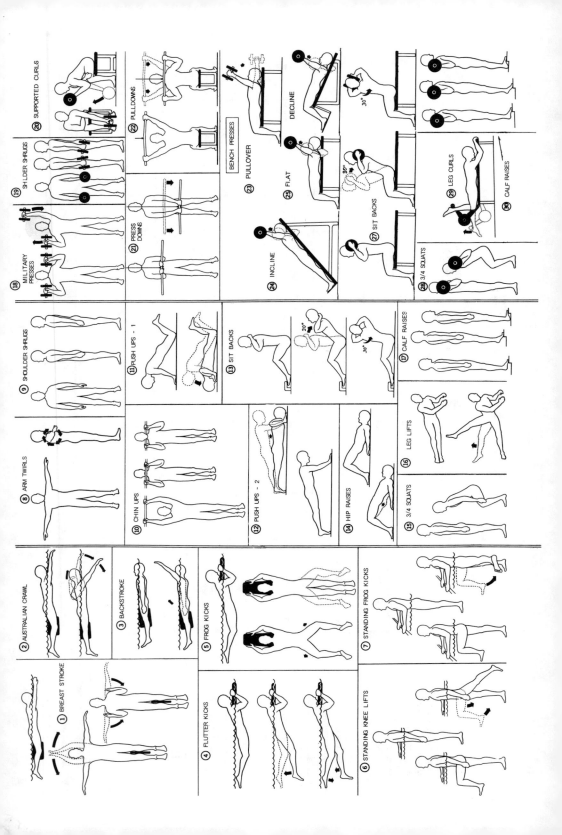

_____'S WORKOUT SCHEDULE FOR _____

(name)   (month)

ACTIVITY	SUNDAY Date / Ck.	MONDAY Date / Ck.	TUESDAY Date / Ck.	WEDNESDAY Date / Ck.	THURSDAY Date / Ck.	FRIDAY Date / Ck.	SATURDAY Date / Ck.

WATER
1. BREAST STROKE
2. AUSTRALIAN CRAWL
3. BACKSTROKE
4. FLUTTER KICKS
5. FROG KICKS
6. STANDING KNEE LIFTS
7. STANDING FROG KICKS

FLOOR
8. ARM TWIRLS
9. SHOULDER SHRUGS
10. CHIN UPS
11. PUSH-UPS - 1
12. PUSH-UPS - 2
13. SIT BACKS
14. HIP RAISES
15. 3/4 SQUATS
16. LEG LIFTS
17. CALF RAISES

WEIGHT ROOM
18. MILITARY PRESSES
WT: _____
RP: _____
19. SHOULDER SHRUGS
WT: _____
RP: _____
20. SUPPORTED CURLS
WT: _____
RP: _____
21. PRESS DOWNS
WT: _____
RP: _____
22. PULLDOWNS
WT: _____
RP: _____
23. FLAT BENCH PULLOVER
WT: _____
RP: _____
24. INCLINE BENCH PRESSES
WT: _____
RP: _____
25. FLAT BENCH PRESSES
WT: _____
RP: _____
26. DECLINE BENCH PRESSES
WT: _____
RP: _____
27. SIT BACKS
WT: _____
RP: _____
28. 3/4 SQUATS
WT: _____
RP: _____
29. LEG CURLS
WT: _____
RP: _____
30. CALF RAISES
WT: _____
RP: _____

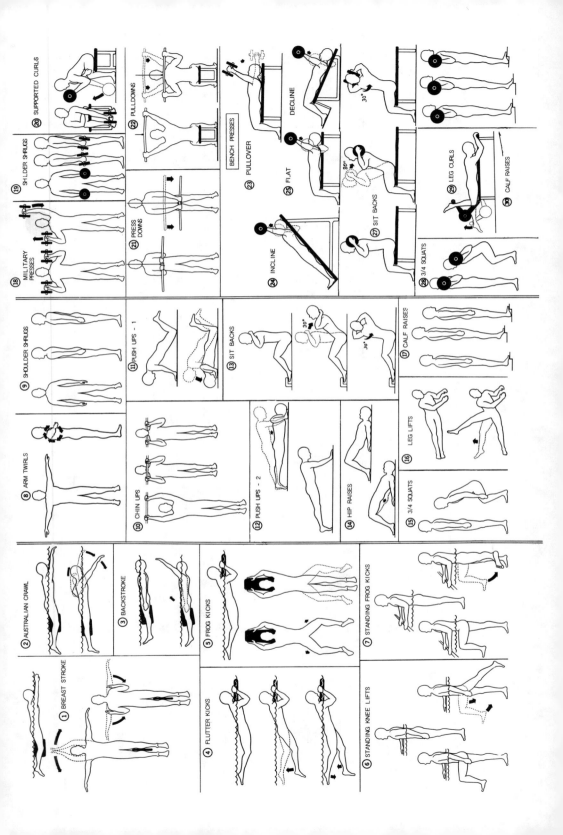

_____'S WORKOUT SCHEDULE FOR _____
(name)   (month)

ACTIVITY	SUNDAY Date / Ck.	MONDAY Date / Ck.	TUESDAY Date / Ck.	WEDNESDAY Date / Ck.	THURSDAY Date / Ck.	FRIDAY Date / Ck.	SATURDAY Date / Ck.

WATER
1. BREAST STROKE
2. AUSTRALIAN CRAWL
3. BACKSTROKE
4. FLUTTER KICKS
5. FROG KICKS
6. STANDING KNEE LIFTS
7. STANDING FROG KICKS

FLOOR
8. ARM TWIRLS
9. SHOULDER SHRUGS
10. CHIN UPS
11. PUSH-UPS - 1
12. PUSH-UPS - 2
13. SIT BACKS
14. HIP RAISES
15. 3/4 SQUATS
16. LEG LIFTS
17. CALF RAISES

WEIGHT ROOM
18. MILITARY PRESSES
    WT:
    RP:
19. SHOULDER SHRUGS
    WT:
    RP:
20. SUPPORTED CURLS
    WT:
    RP:
21. PRESS DOWNS
    WT:
    RP:
22. PULLDOWNS
    WT:
    RP:
23. FLAT BENCH PULLOVER
    WT:
    RP:
24. INCLINE BENCH PRESSES
    WT:
    RP:
25. FLAT BENCH PRESSES
    WT:
    RP:
26. DECLINE BENCH PRESSES
    WT:
    RP:
27. SIT BACKS
    WT:
    RP:
28. 3/4 SQUATS
    WT:
    RP:
29. LEG CURLS
    WT:
    RP:
30. CALF RAISES
    WT:
    RP:

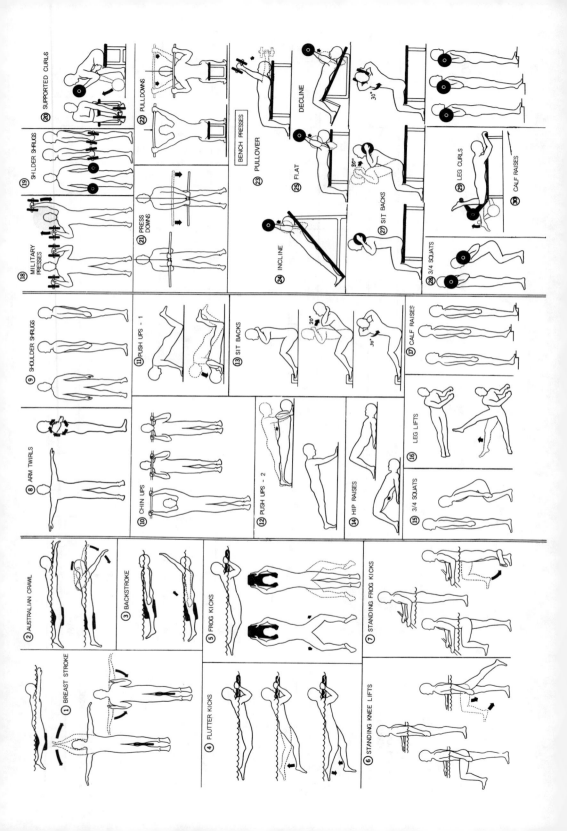

_____'S WORKOUT SCHEDULE FOR _____
(name)   (month)

ACTIVITY

WATER
1. BREAST STROKE
2. AUSTRALIAN CRAWL
3. BACKSTROKE
4. FLUTTER KICKS
5. FROG KICKS
6. STANDING KNEE LIFTS
7. STANDING FROG KICKS

FLOOR
8. ARM TWIRLS
9. SHOULDER SHRUGS
10. CHIN UPS
11. PUSH-UPS - 1
12. PUSH-UPS - 2
13. SIT BACKS
14. HIP RAISES
15. 3/4 SQUATS
16. LEG LIFTS
17. CALF RAISES

WEIGHT ROOM

18. MILITARY PRESSES
    WT:
    RP:
19. SHOULDER SHRUGS
    WT:
    RP:
20. SUPPORTED CURLS
    WT:
    RP:
21. PRESS DOWNS
    WT:
    RP:
22. PULLDOWNS
    WT:
    RP:
23. FLAT BENCH PULLOVER
    WT:
    RP:
24. INCLINE BENCH PRESSES
    WT:
    RP:
25. FLAT BENCH PRESSES
    WT:
    RP:
26. DECLINE BENCH PRESSES
    WT:
    RP:
27. SIT BACKS
    WT:
    RP:
28. 3/4 SQUATS
    WT:
    RP:
29. LEG CURLS
    WT:
    RP:
30. CALF RAISES
    WT:
    RP:

	SUNDAY Date / Ck.	MONDAY Date / Ck.	TUESDAY Date / Ck.	WEDNESDAY Date / Ck.	THURSDAY Date / Ck.	FRIDAY Date / Ck.	SATURDAY Date / Ck.

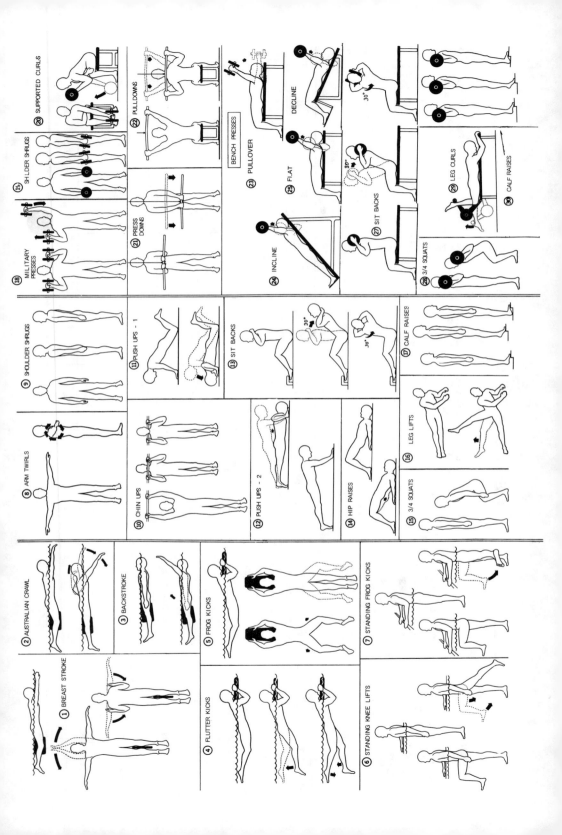

_____'S WORKOUT SCHEDULE FOR _____

(name) (month)

ACTIVITY

WATER
1. BREAST STROKE
2. AUSTRALIAN CRAWL
3. BACKSTROKE
4. FLUTTER KICKS
5. FROG KICKS
6. STANDING KNEE LIFTS
7. STANDING FROG KICKS

FLOOR
8. ARM TWIRLS
9. SHOULDER SHRUGS
10. CHIN UPS
11. PUSH-UPS - 1
12. PUSH-UPS - 2
13. SIT BACKS
14. HIP RAISES
15. 3/4 SQUATS
16. LEG LIFTS
17. CALF RAISES

WEIGHT ROOM

18. MILITARY PRESSES
   WT:
   RP:

19. SHOULDER SHRUGS
   WT:
   RP:

20. SUPPORTED CURLS
   WT:
   RP:

21. PRESS DOWNS
   WT:
   RP:

22. PULLDOWNS
   WT:
   RP:

23. FLAT BENCH PULLOVER
   WT:
   RP:

24. INCLINE BENCH PRESSES
   WT:
   RP:

25. FLAT BENCH PRESSES
   WT:
   RP:

26. DECLINE BENCH PRESSES
   WT:
   RP:

27. SIT BACKS
   WT:
   RP:

28. 3/4 SQUATS
   WT:
   RP:

29. LEG CURLS
   WT:
   RP:

30. CALF RAISES
   WT:
   RP:

	SUNDAY Date / Ck.	MONDAY Date / Ck.	TUESDAY Date / Ck.	WEDNESDAY Date / Ck.	THURSDAY Date / Ck.	FRIDAY Date / Ck.	SATURDAY Date / Ck.

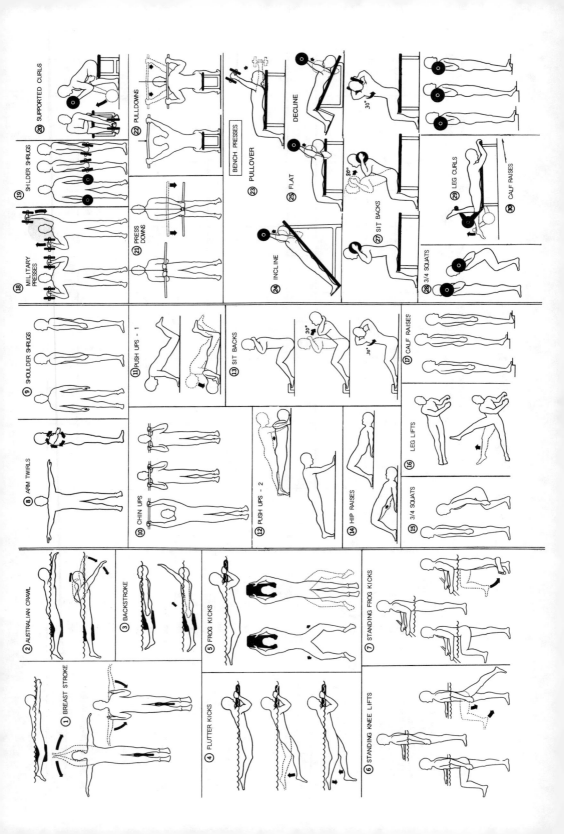

_____'s WORKOUT SCHEDULE FOR _____

(name) (month)

ACTIVITY	SUNDAY Date / Ck.	MONDAY Date / Ck.	TUESDAY Date / Ck.	WEDNESDAY Date / Ck.	THURSDAY Date / Ck.	FRIDAY Date / Ck.	SATURDAY Date / Ck.
WATER							
1 BREAST STROKE							
2 AUSTRALIAN CRAWL							
3 BACKSTROKE							
4 FLUTTER KICKS							
5 FROG KICKS							
6 STANDING KNEE LIFTS							
7 STANDING FROG KICKS							
FLOOR							
8 ARM TWIRLS							
9 SHOULDER SHRUGS							
10 CHIN UPS							
11 PUSH-UPS - 1							
12 PUSH-UPS - 2							
13 SIT BACKS							
14 HIP RAISES							
15 3/4 SQUATS							
16 LEG LIFTS							
17 CALF RAISES							

WEIGHT ROOM

18 MILITARY PRESSES WT: / RP:							
19 SHOULDER SHRUGS WT: / RP:							
20 SUPPORTED CURLS WT: / RP:							
21 PRESS DOWNS WT: / RP:							
22 PULLDOWNS WT: / RP:							
23 FLAT BENCH PULLOVER WT: / RP:							
24 INCLINE BENCH PRESSES WT: / RP:							
25 FLAT BENCH PRESSES WT: / RP:							
26 DECLINE BENCH PRESSES WT: / RP:							
27 SIT BACKS WT: / RP:							
28 3/4 SQUATS WT: / RP:							
29 LEG CURLS WT: / RP:							
30 CALF RAISES WT: / RP:							

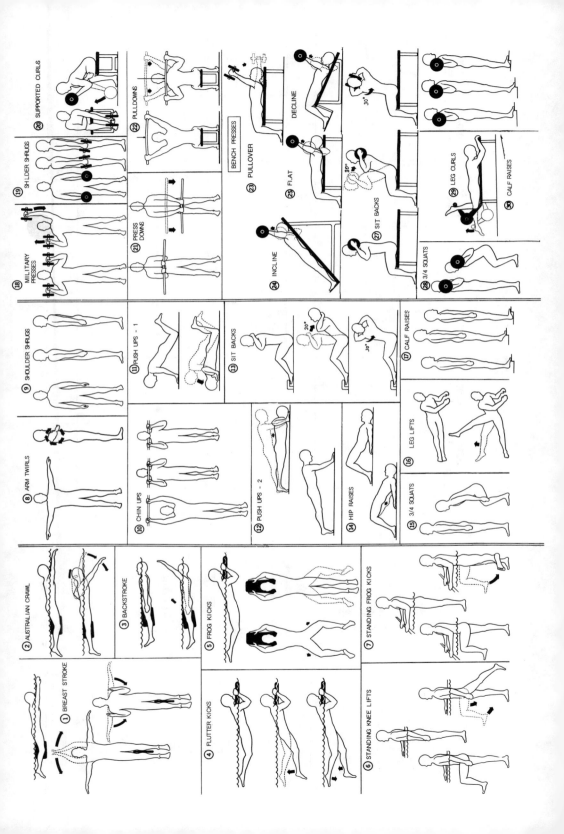

_____'S WORKOUT SCHEDULE FOR _____ (month)

(name)

ACTIVITY	SUNDAY Date / Ck.	MONDAY Date / Ck.	TUESDAY Date / Ck.	WEDNESDAY Date / Ck.	THURSDAY Date / Ck.	FRIDAY Date / Ck.	SATURDAY Date / Ck.

WATER
1. BREAST STROKE
2. AUSTRALIAN CRAWL
3. BACKSTROKE
4. FLUTTER KICKS
5. FROG KICKS
6. STANDING KNEE LIFTS
7. STANDING FROG KICKS

FLOOR
8. ARM TWIRLS
9. SHOULDER SHRUGS
10. CHIN UPS
11. PUSH-UPS - 1
12. PUSH-UPS - 2
13. SIT BACKS
14. HIP RAISES
15. 3/4 SQUATS
16. LEG LIFTS
17. CALF RAISES

WEIGHT ROOM

18. MILITARY PRESSES
   WT: ___
   RP: ___

19. SHOULDER SHRUGS
   WT: ___
   RP: ___

20. SUPPORTED CURLS
   WT: ___
   RP: ___

21. PRESS DOWNS
   WT: ___
   RP: ___

22. PULLDOWNS
   WT: ___
   RP: ___

23. FLAT BENCH PULLOVER
   WT: ___
   RP: ___

24. INCLINE BENCH PRESSES
   WT: ___
   RP: ___

25. FLAT BENCH PRESSES
   WT: ___
   RP: ___

26. DECLINE BENCH PRESSES
   WT: ___
   RP: ___

27. SIT BACKS
   WT: ___
   RP: ___

28. 3/4 SQUATS
   WT: ___
   RP: ___

29. LEG CURLS
   WT: ___
   RP: ___

30. CALF RAISES
   WT: ___
   RP: ___

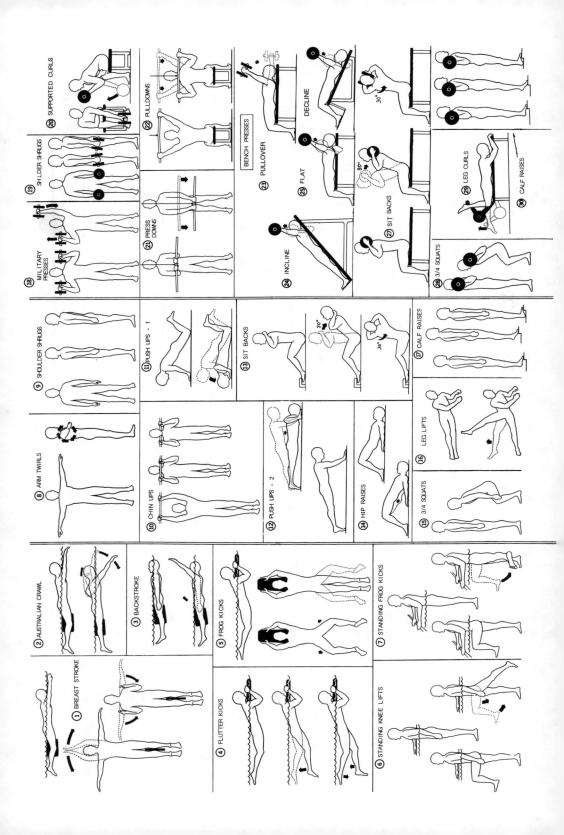

_____'s WORKOUT SCHEDULE FOR _____
(name)   (month)

ACTIVITY	SUNDAY Date / Ck.	MONDAY Date / Ck.	TUESDAY Date / Ck.	WEDNESDAY Date / Ck.	THURSDAY Date / Ck.	FRIDAY Date / Ck.	SATURDAY Date / Ck.

ACTIVITY

WATER
1. BREAST STROKE
2. AUSTRALIAN CRAWL
3. BACKSTROKE
4. FLUTTER KICKS
5. FROG KICKS
6. STANDING KNEE LIFTS
7. STANDING FROG KICKS

FLOOR
8. ARM TWIRLS
9. SHOULDER SHRUGS
10. CHIN UPS
11. PUSH-UPS - 1
12. PUSH-UPS - 2
13. SIT BACKS
14. HIP RAISES
15. 3/4 SQUATS
16. LEG LIFTS
17. CALF RAISES

WEIGHT ROOM
18. MILITARY PRESSES
    WT:
    RP:
19. SHOULDER SHRUGS
    WT:
    RP:
20. SUPPORTED CURLS
    WT:
    RP:
21. PRESS DOWNS
    WT:
    RP:
22. PULLDOWNS
    WT:
    RP:
23. FLAT BENCH PULLOVER
    WT:
    RP:
24. INCLINE BENCH PRESSES
    WT:
    RP:
25. FLAT BENCH PRESSES
    WT:
    RP:
26. DECLINE BENCH PRESSES
    WT:
    RP:
27. SIT BACKS
    WT:
    RP:
28. 3/4 SQUATS
    WT:
    RP:
29. LEG CURLS
    WT:
    RP:
30. CALF RAISES
    WT:
    RP:

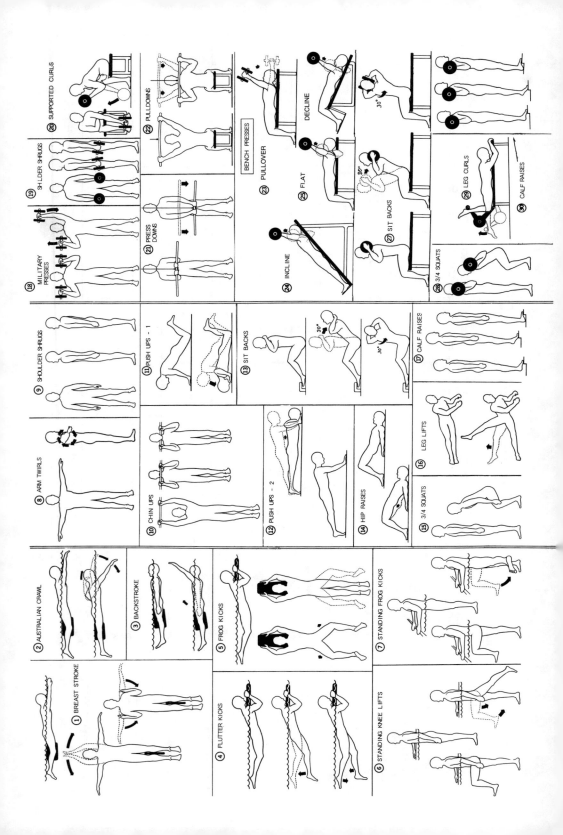

_____'S WORKOUT SCHEDULE FOR _____
(name)   (month)

ACTIVITY

WATER
1. BREAST STROKE
2. AUSTRALIAN CRAWL
3. BACKSTROKE
4. FLUTTER KICKS
5. FROG KICKS
6. STANDING KNEE LIFTS
7. STANDING FROG KICKS

FLOOR
8. ARM TWIRLS
9. SHOULDER SHRUGS
10. CHIN UPS
11. PUSH-UPS - 1
12. PUSH-UPS - 2
13. SIT BACKS
14. HIP RAISES
15. 3/4 SQUATS
16. LEG LIFTS
17. CALF RAISES

WEIGHT ROOM

18. MILITARY PRESSES
    WT:
    RP:
19. SHOULDER SHRUGS
    WT:
    RP:
20. SUPPORTED CURLS
    WT:
    RP:
21. PRESS DOWNS
    WT:
    RP:
22. PULLDOWNS
    WT:
    RP:
23. FLAT BENCH PULLOVER
    WT:
    RP:
24. INCLINE BENCH PRESSES
    WT:
    RP:
25. FLAT BENCH PRESSES
    WT:
    RP:
26. DECLINE BENCH PRESSES
    WT:
    RP:
27. SIT BACKS
    WT:
    RP:
28. 3/4 SQUATS
    WT:
    RP:
29. LEG CURLS
    WT:
    RP:
30. CALF RAISES
    WT:
    RP:

	SUNDAY Date / Ck.	MONDAY Date / Ck.	TUESDAY Date / Ck.	WEDNESDAY Date / Ck.	THURSDAY Date / Ck.	FRIDAY Date / Ck.	SATURDAY Date / Ck.

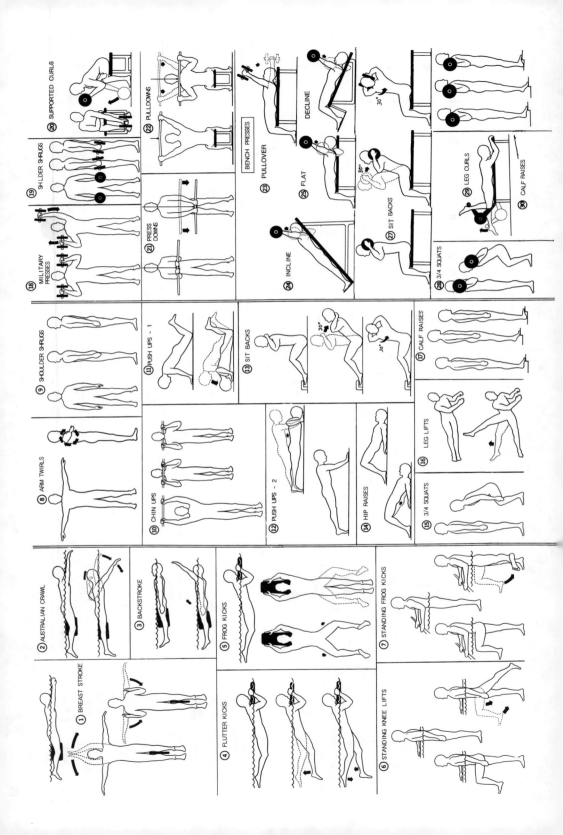

_____'S WORKOUT SCHEDULE FOR _____

(name)   (month)

ACTIVITY

WATER
1. BREAST STROKE
2. AUSTRALIAN CRAWL
3. BACKSTROKE
4. FLUTTER KICKS
5. FROG KICKS
6. STANDING KNEE LIFTS
7. STANDING FROG KICKS

FLOOR
8. ARM TWIRLS
9. SHOULDER SHRUGS
10. CHIN UPS
11. PUSH-UPS - 1
12. PUSH-UPS - 2
13. SIT BACKS
14. HIP RAISES
15. 3/4 SQUATS
16. LEG LIFTS
17. CALF RAISES

WEIGHT ROOM

18. MILITARY PRESSES
WT:
RP:

19. SHOULDER SHRUGS
WT:
RP:

20. SUPPORTED CURLS
WT:
RP:

21. PRESS DOWNS
WT:
RP:

22. PULLDOWNS
WT:
RP:

23. FLAT BENCH PULLOVER
WT:
RP:

24. INCLINE BENCH PRESSES
WT:
RP:

25. FLAT BENCH PRESSES
WT:
RP:

26. DECLINE BENCH PRESSES
WT:
RP:

27. SIT BACKS
WT:
RP:

28. 3/4 SQUATS
WT:
RP:

29. LEG CURLS
WT:
RP:

30. CALF RAISES
WT:
RP:

	SUNDAY Date / Ck.	MONDAY Date / Ck.	TUESDAY Date / Ck.	WEDNESDAY Date / Ck.	THURSDAY Date / Ck.	FRIDAY Date / Ck.	SATURDAY Date / Ck.

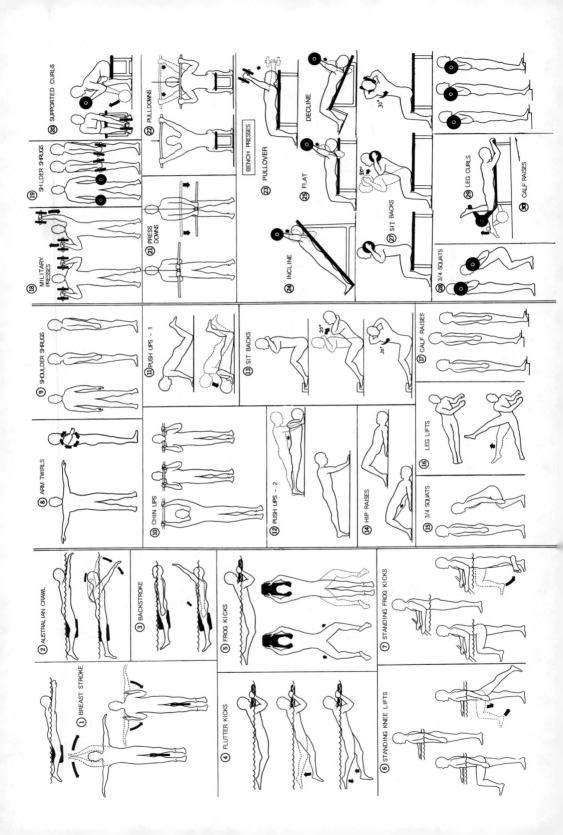

_____'S WORKOUT SCHEDULE FOR _____

(name)   (month)

ACTIVITY

WATER
1. BREAST STROKE
2. AUSTRALIAN CRAWL
3. BACKSTROKE
4. FLUTTER KICKS
5. FROG KICKS
6. STANDING KNEE LIFTS
7. STANDING FROG KICKS

FLOOR
8. ARM TWIRLS
9. SHOULDER SHRUGS
10. CHIN UPS
11. PUSH-UPS - 1
12. PUSH-UPS - 2
13. SIT BACKS
14. HIP RAISES
15. 3/4 SQUATS
16. LEG LIFTS
17. CALF RAISES

WEIGHT ROOM
18. MILITARY PRESSES — WT: ___ RP: ___
19. SHOULDER SHRUGS — WT: ___ RP: ___
20. SUPPORTED CURLS — WT: ___ RP: ___
21. PRESS DOWNS — WT: ___ RP: ___
22. PULLDOWNS — WT: ___ RP: ___
23. FLAT BENCH PULLOVER — WT: ___ RP: ___
24. INCLINE BENCH PRESSES — WT: ___ RP: ___
25. FLAT BENCH PRESSES — WT: ___ RP: ___
26. DECLINE BENCH PRESSES — WT: ___ RP: ___
27. SIT BACKS — WT: ___ RP: ___
28. 3/4 SQUATS — WT: ___ RP: ___
29. LEG CURLS — WT: ___ RP: ___
30. CALF RAISES — WT: ___ RP: ___

	SUNDAY Date / Ck.	MONDAY Date / Ck.	TUESDAY Date / Ck.	WEDNESDAY Date / Ck.	THURSDAY Date / Ck.	FRIDAY Date / Ck.	SATURDAY Date / Ck.

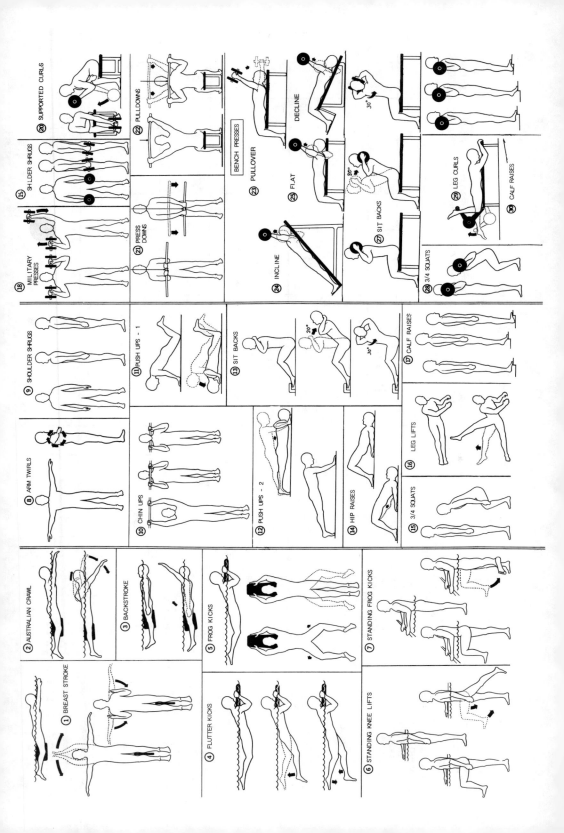

_____'S WORKOUT SCHEDULE FOR _____

(name)   (month)

ACTIVITY	SUNDAY Date / Ck.	MONDAY Date / Ck.	TUESDAY Date / Ck.	WEDNESDAY Date / Ck.	THURSDAY Date / Ck.	FRIDAY Date / Ck.	SATURDAY Date / Ck.
WATER							
1 BREAST STROKE							
2 AUSTRALIAN CRAWL							
3 BACKSTROKE							
4 FLUTTER KICKS							
5 FROG KICKS							
6 STANDING KNEE LIFTS							
7 STANDING FROG KICKS							
FLOOR							
8 ARM TWIRLS							
9 SHOULDER SHRUGS							
10 CHIN UPS							
11 PUSH-UPS - 1							
12 PUSH-UPS - 2							
13 SIT BACKS							
14 HIP RAISES							
15 3/4 SQUATS							
16 LEG LIFTS							
17 CALF RAISES							
WEIGHT ROOM							
18 MILITARY PRESSES WT: RP:							
19 SHOULDER SHRUGS WT: RP:							
20 SUPPORTED CURLS WT: RP:							
21 PRESS DOWNS WT: RP:							
22 PULLDOWNS WT: RP:							
23 FLAT BENCH PULLOVER WT: RP:							
24 INCLINE BENCH PRESSES WT: RP:							
25 FLAT BENCH PRESSES WT: RP:							
26 DECLINE BENCH PRESSES WT: RP:							
27 SIT BACKS WT: RP:							
28 3/4 SQUATS WT: RP:							
29 LEG CURLS WT: RP:							
30 CALF RAISES WT: RP:							

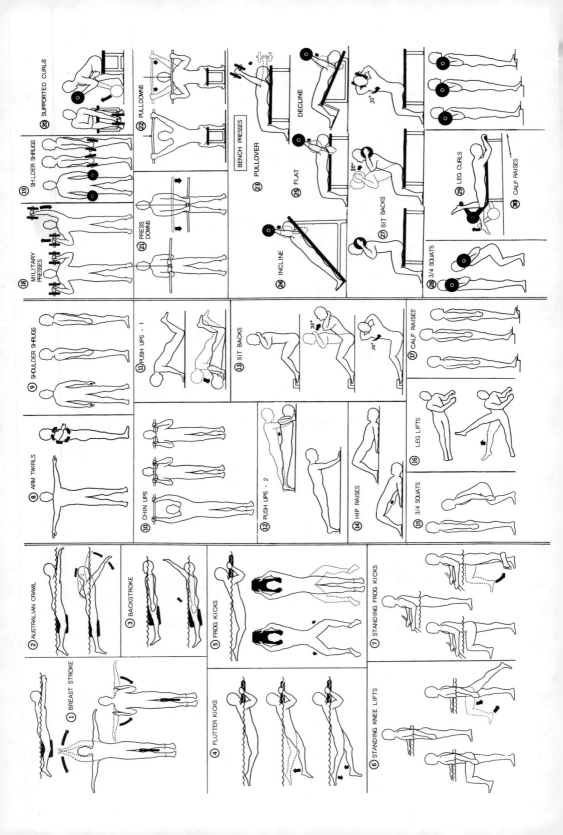